Triumph

ENDORSEMENTS

"*Triumph* is a fitting title for this raw reflection on Greg's journey. I can attest to some of the unvarnished truth and wisdom he shares in *Triumph*. I believe God built us for community, for each other. Community not only helps us with our challenges but helps us focus on God as our true source and provider. It amazes me how even though Greg was going through an enormous challenge, he still took time to invest in others. Greg's investment in others allowed God to shower him with blessings that contributed to his healing and recovery."

Hollis Williams
Chief Executive Officer, EKI-Digital

"Greg took on the challenge of dealing with a potentially debilitating illness, polycystic kidney disease. He conquered kidney disease by committing to the lifestyle changes that preserved his life and allowed him to inspire others. Sometimes God does something *to* you, to do something *for* you. Greg showed valor, humility, and strength, as an example for his family and others, to witness, in real time, strategies for pushing through adversity. *Triumph* inspired me, and I know it will inspire so many others."

Dimitrius Hutcherson
Executive Vice President, First Independence Bank

"*Triumph* is a must-read that describes how to battle a health crisis while facing menacing medical trials, financial uncertainty, spiritual certainty and the unknown. Watch Greg's faith prevail as he slays medical giants not once, but twice. The principles he outlines are applicable for effectively combating kidney disease, cancer, diabetes, and other life altering medical conditions. Greg's courage and optimism permit him to lean on God as the source of his strength and persistence."

Frank Dyer
Chief Operating Officer, T.D. Jakes Ministries

"This captivating read is part memoir, part instructional manual on how to be a successful organ transplant recipient. It provides a blueprint for navigating the harrowing experience of becoming an organ recipient and nurturing the fragile nature of life. In *Triumph*, we learn how faith, redemption, the power of prayer, and obedience serve as building blocks that let us bear witness to the mesmerizing manner in which God works miracles for those who love Him."

Norma L. Day-Vines, Ph.D.
Interim Vice Dean, Academic Affairs, Associate Dean, Diversity and Faculty Development, Professor, Counseling and Educational Studies, Johns Hopkins University

"This is a brilliant original work. Greg provides a thoughtful and detailed process for managing a chronic and often fatal disease such as polycystic kidney disease. He used his faith, family, fortitude, and the instructions of his medical team as his compass. Triumph provides a roadmap for anyone facing a major medical condition, personal angst and debilitating depression. *Triumph* is your guide to clarity, diligence, and serenity in the face of life-threatening disease!"

Kannan Sreedhar
(Retired) General Manager, Vice President, Avaya

"*Triumph* gives readers a front row seat to Greg's health challenges as his faith transitions from "water skiing" to "scuba diving" based on his trust in God. Greg bravely reframes his suffering and sees it as his calling to bring optimism to others facing adversity. Get ready to be injected with hope in your obstacles."

Dr. Johnny Parker

Director of 10x Better Man First Baptist Church of Glenarden

Author of *Turn the Page: Unlocking the Story Within You*

TRIUMPH

Life on the Other Side
of Trials, Transplants,
Transition and Transformation

GREGORY S. WORKS

NEW YORK

LONDON • NASHVILLE • MELBOURNE • VANCOUVER

Triumph

Life on the Other Side of Trials, Transplants, Transition, and Transformation

Published in New York, New York, by Morgan James Publishing. Morgan James is a trademark of Morgan James, LLC. www.MorganJamesPublishing.com

Proudly distributed by Publishers Group West®

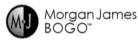

ISBN 9781636980621 paperback
ISBN 9781636980638 ebook
Library of Congress Control Number: 2022945986

Cover Design by:
Rachel Lopez
www.r2cdesign.com

Interior Design by:
Christopher Kirk
www.GFSstudio.com

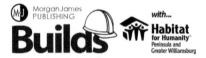

Morgan James is a proud partner of Habitat for Humanity Peninsula and Greater Williamsburg. Partners in building since 2006.

Get involved today! Visit: www.morgan-james-publishing.com/giving-back

To my parents, Bobby and Nancy Works, who encouraged me to tell this story which impacted everyone in our immediate family (including my sisters, Sharon and Kharon). To my wife Cynthia, and daughter's, Kylie and Kelsey for your support, patience, and care. You have had a front-row seat watching my battle fighting Polycystic Kidney Disease, and I pray that I am the last to encounter this battle from our immediate family.

TABLE OF CONTENTS

ACKNOWLEDGMENTS

A project like this doesn't emerge unless there is a community of individuals committed its execution. I must thank David Hancock, founder of Morgan James Publishing, for his enthusiasm, patience and desire to want to help tell this story. You opened my eyes to audiences this story can impact that I never considered. I owe a debt of gratitude to Raoul Davis, president of The Ascendant Group, for providing the Team to assist me in writing, branding and marketing *Triumph*. You understood the story I was telling and what could make it stand out in a crowd of books focused on hope, overcoming, and transformation following a major challenge. To my writers and editors, Rainah Davis and Tiara Brown, I am eternally grateful because you spent countless hours with me gaining a firsthand account of how I overcame obstacles, highlighting faith as a foundation to triumph, and talking to significant others that helped me along the way. Steve Pemberton, author, motivational speaker and Chief People Officer for Workhuman, I appreciate you for listening to my story and believing it was compelling and worthy of being told. You helped me turn my story into a reality that can inspire people across the globe. To Kevin DaSilva, thank you for encouraging me to share my story with a group of friends and family over lunch and introducing me to Steve Pemberton.

I would like to especially thank my wife, Cynthia and daughters, Kylie and Kelsey for your love and support and for giving me the space I needed to put my story in writing and undertake such an important project. I only wish there was a similar book for me to read to help me along my transplant journey. To my parents, Nancy and Bobby Works, who are no longer with us, thank you for preparing me for this journey and helping me see that my illness had a purpose, and for seeing the good that could transpire in the midst of the challenge. To Sharon and Kharon, my sisters, I send my gratitude for your unwavering support and having a shoulder to lean on. Special thanks to my BID (Brothers In Discipleship) brother, Vaughn Johnson, for praying with me several times a week. Your support grounded me and helped me believe my breakthrough was always right around the corner. To my kidney donors, William Snoddy, as well as Dave and Kristen Seagar, I am grateful to you for providing me the gift that keeps on giving. Your donations have extended my life. Thank you to my family and close friends, far too many to name, that supported and prayed for me and my family throughout this journey. Above all, I would like to thank my Lord and Savior, Jesus Christ, for walking with me every step of the way and producing miracles that showed He and only He could orchestrate the triumphs that were happening.

FOREWORD

We hopefully find many lessons that contributed to our faith and personal development when we focus on the events, challenges, and opportunities that presented themselves in 2022 (and its preceding couple of years). Those who emerged wiser, more enlightened, and more fortified for the future are the ones who sought inspiration, motivation, and empathy in their personal experiences and observations of others. By writing Triumph, Greg Works taps into his legacy as a father, son, family member, and businessman. As an excellent Christian steward, he successfully transforms his personal challenges into a rewarding testimony that benefits others.

Whether or not you or a family member are dealing with kidney disease, Triumph is a compelling read because it details a man's commitment to his family and friends. This book also describes how one can successfully marshal the resources at their disposal to overcome adversity with a positive attitude. We all have or will face challenges that knock us off balance and test our faith. Triumph is a tool we can utilize to fortify ourselves to stay the course and encourage those battling with us.

Greg Works' frequent references to his faith, children, wife, sisters, father, mother, and friends reflect his values and motivation for authoring Triumph. As he continues his battle with kidney disease, he continues learning and teaching, and readers reap those benefits. As I watched Greg in his health journey, he never lost his faith or sense of humor. He always believed he would receive the kidneys he needed for his transplants and remained intentional about caring for those who accompanied him on his journey. Similarly, as he dealt with the loss of his parents to kidney disease, Greg shared a testimony about how his parents inspired and supported him throughout his battles with PKD. As a result, the theme of family is woven throughout Triumph, highlighted by Greg's difficult decision to accept dialysis as a solution (after his mother's unfortunate experience).

I was not surprised to read Greg's description of the character traits that bolstered his survival because these are traits those close to Greg have witnessed in his life for years. His strong and unyielding faith in God, perseverance, refusal to accept failure, and determination to use his platform to publish his testimony, are similar to his propensity to launch and extend a conversation. If among the qualifications for an author is the ability to tell a story, then Greg Works is inarguably the man for the job. Triumph reads like a conversation with Greg; if you ever have that pleasure, you will be entertained, enlightened, and late for your next appointment!

If you ask Greg why he wrote Triumph, he will share that he knew he would have benefited from this kind of book at the beginning of his challenges. Triumph is a talk with a friend who has successfully dealt with difficulties associated with kidney disease, gleaned insights from his family's struggles with the same illness, and is duty-bound to articulate the tips he learned along the way. His approach reflects his academic background, sales experience, business expertise, and Bible study methods such as: praying (segment obstacles and don't let them overwhelm you), listening (and following directions), developing (a game plan and being intentional), being humble, being prepared for detours (and rocky roads), understanding constraints, and believing in the impossible. Ultimately, Greg provides a roadmap for those whose journey follows his. The benefits of Triumph apply to a broad target audience, extending beyond those managing illnesses to medical professionals, clergy, millennials and younger audiences, and those dealing with extreme crises or challenges.

Furthermore, as kidney diseases have genetically and circumstantially been pervasive in Greg Works' family, these virtues have been manifested in their lives, and the legacies passed on to their children. When I recently attended the memorial services for Bobby Works, Greg's father, and mentor, I was reminded of the Works' family model: fatherhood, "covering" your family (another Greg Works classic), demonstrating faith, and supporting others through their trials. To his family's credit, these services expanded to serve many purposes, including highlighting virtues that inspire others.

My exposure to Greg and his family for more than 30 years and my parallel exposure to transplant medicine as a health care professional provide me with a unique perspective. I empathize with those who have wrestled with life-altering circumstances and would benefit from the inspiration and insights in Triumph—especially because experiencing a kidney transplant is noteworthy. While kidney diseases are common, because of the lack of availability of transplant organs, not many of us know someone close to us who has had one or more surgeries. Greg's story of faith includes the curse of kidney disease and the blessing of multiple transplants.

Ultimately, this book is required reading because Greg details his version of triumph, faith, family, and friendship. I have been privileged and blessed to be a part of Greg's circle of friends—one that ranks among the broadest I have encountered. By reading Triumph, you will also join that fortunate circle. It has been said that "one who has a broad circle of friends must himself be friendly." Triumph illustrates testimonies articulated by someone who has been *through the fire* and is *on fire* to share knowledge that will serve others.

Unfortunately, heartbreaking stories of kidney disease are becoming more common, and testimonies about the battle against this disease are multiplying. An internet search for books on the topic yielded more than 200 responses before I stopped scrolling down and realized I had made my point. In this crowded genre, a book about faith over fear, leading an empowered life, and adopting a triumphant attitude stands out. Greg Works' circumstances are not unique. His approach to his circumstances, determination to overcome a debilitating disease, and testimony about his success in continuing to live a wholesome and committed life are unique and inspiring. In addition to medical treatments and transplants, those suffering from PKD need encouragement, inspiration, and advice. Greg knows this well and uses his unique communication style and practical sales skills to provide insight to patients, their supportive families, and potential organ donors.

—Herbert Buchanan
Senior Vice President and Chief Operating Officer
Great Lakes Region, AdventHealth

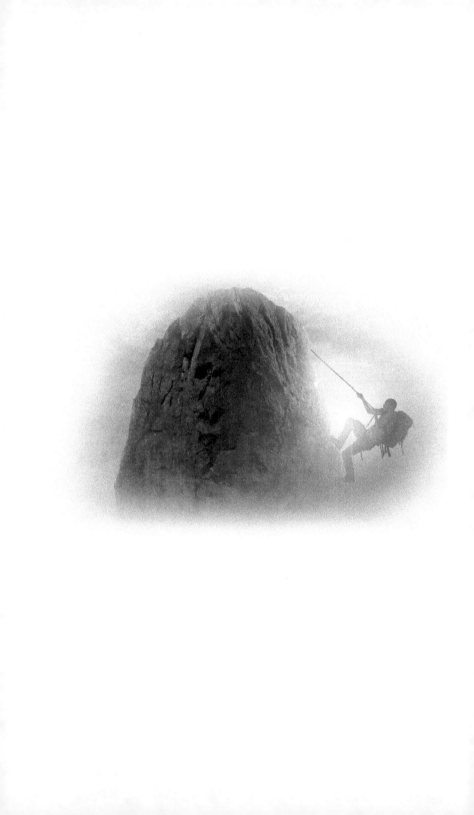

PART 1
MY TESTIMONY

Chapter 1

AN UNEXPECTED DISCOVERY

As I pen the words to this book, our country has been turned upside down, and chaos has broken out, not just within our nation but globally as well. Many things, consequently, will be forever changed in the wake of the COVID-19 pandemic. Individuals most vulnerable to COVID-19 have undergone a complete change and therefore had to eliminate things they enjoy most. I can relate to that necessity because I am in that group; my life changed dramatically many years ago.

Memory Lane

As my mind treads down memory lane, I fondly recall a challenge that was made to me that, if accepted, would become a regular facet of my life. I lived in the Washington, DC, Metropolitan Area at the time. The challenge was to go to the University of Maryland and run the stairs at SECU Stadium (formerly known as Capital One Field at Maryland Stadium). The joke was that if I did not accept the challenge, one day, I would grow to become fat, old, and bald. I responded by accepting the challenge. Running the stairs may not sound like a feat, but it was after I attempted the workout myself.

In the summer of 2004, I began driving to the University of Maryland, meeting with a group of friends, and running the stadium stairs. This high-intensity workout was the most intense exercise regimen I have ever experienced. It worked on cardio, endurance, and balance, and strengthened my lower leg muscles. Running the stairs impacted every fabric of my being, which was great; however, the camaraderie and competition were even better. During that time, my friends and I laughed and shared stories about the general stresses of life:

- Work-life balance
- Being good husbands
- Getting ahead in our respective careers

There was not much work-life balance at that time in my career. I worked in business development for a Big Four consulting firm that recently transitioned from a privately held company to a publicly traded company. The pressure to perform was intense. My role was to generate new business, expand all existing business, establish new client relationships, and develop new and existing partner relationships. While my focus was to perform, the company was experiencing increasing resource, process, and financial challenges while transitioning to a publicly traded company. As a result, these challenges directly impacted my ability to win new business. It was the perfect storm. Constantly living under this Damoclean sword while pursuing multimillion-dollar deals was beginning to take a toll on me.

I remember an article on the front page of the business section of The Washington Post. The feature highlighted the financial challenges my company was experiencing and reiterated the dangers associated with the organization's future. The purport of this article created significant anxiety for me, and I was not optimistic about what was to come.

My Annual Physical

In the fall of 2004, I scheduled my annual physical with my primary care physician (PCP). I had been using this PCP for at least six years. He was very aware of my medical history and that of my family. Even though my parents and siblings did not use his medical services, he knew some ailments and diseases were hereditary that could be passed down and impact me directly.

As scheduled, I went into the medical office to have my physical. Everything went as planned. The doctor conducted a thorough examination. He checked my height, weight, blood pressure, and eyes, performed an electrocardiogram (EKG), conducted a prostate examination, and drew blood. Everything appeared to go as well as could be expected. Externally, nothing was alarming, and there were no signs of illness. A few days after my appointment, my PCP called to share my lab results. Based on my results, my doctor sent me to a specialist to take some additional tests and x-rays. He was concerned because some numbers were elevated, and he wanted to gain a better understanding to provide the best diagnosis to treat any ailments that may arise.

A couple of days later, I received a call from my PCP. He shared that the X-rays revealed there were small cysts surrounding my kidneys. Naturally, the phone call and subsequent news caught me off guard. I knew something was wrong. Without hesitation, the doctor said I had Polycystic Kidney Disease.

PKD

Polycystic Kidney Disease, or PKD as it is commonly called, is a genetic disorder that causes many fluid-filled cysts to grow in your kidneys. Unlike the usually harmless cysts that can form in the kidneys later in life, PKD cysts can change the shape of your kidneys (making them larger). PKD is a form of chronic kidney disease (CKD) that reduces kidney function and may lead to kidney failure. PKD also can cause other complications or problems, such as high blood pressure, cysts in the liver, and problems with blood vessels in your brain and heart.

There is no cure for Polycystic Kidney Disease. Doctors have shared that people with PKD must keep themselves hydrated; drinking as much water as possible is very important. One should refrain from all caffeine. Beverages such as coffee, tea, soda, and food made with caffeine can cause a major strain on the kidneys.

Family History

Upon receiving the PKD diagnosis and learning about the disease, I grew to understand that my high blood pressure was directly related to PKD—one of its many symptoms and the reason I was taking blood pressure medications. For over ten years, I wondered why I had high blood pressure. I played sports throughout high school and worked out consistently into adulthood. I always had high-pressure jobs, so stress was a significant factor. My diet was questionable (given I liked to eat at fast-food restaurants); however, the doctors could not pinpoint the source of my high blood pressure. Instead, they shared that it was probably hereditary because it was a common ailment my parents endured. But I needed to know more.

PKD is hereditary on my mother's side of the family. My maternal grandmother was diagnosed, and she passed this disease down to her children (my uncle and my mother). Of the five grandchildren that were conceived from my maternal grandmother's children (three in my family and two in my uncle's family), my sisters and I have PKD, and there is a fair chance the other two grandchildren inherited it as well. Every child conceived from the union of Bobby and Nancy Works was diagnosed with PKD by the age of forty and eventually treated with a kidney transplant. In addition, one of my first cousins had a kidney transplant a few years ago. I was the first of the Works children to need a transplant. My sisters began experiencing symptoms from PKD and subsequently had kidney transplants fourteen months apart from one another during the COVID-19 pandemic.

PKD has significantly impacted my family and the need to treat it through transplants. My mother was diagnosed in her mid-forties and was monitored for kidney disease for years. In her early sixties, she went on dialysis to enhance her kidney functionality. She had been on dialysis for less than a year when she received a call one evening that a kidney became available off the kidney transplant list. The following morning, my sisters and I met our parents at the hospital for my mother's kidney transplant.

My mother's kidney transplant was successful. She moved around with ease post-transplant and was truly living a normal life. The transplanted kidney did well for many years. However, after about eight years, we began to see a decline in her kidney functionality. Her medical team continuously monitored her. She later learned that a virus was attacking her kidney. It got to the point where her doctors said they would need to remove the kidney, or the virus could take her life. So, after much thought, prayer and consultation, it was recommended that surgery be scheduled. The kidney was eventually removed, and my mother went back on dialysis.

About a year later, my mother underwent routine dialysis treatment. One day, upon completion of a dialysis exchange, my mother stood up and collapsed—her heart stopped beating. The nurses, doctors, and specialists worked to revive her, but to no avail; we lost her. That tragic episode took place in January 2013. Not a day goes by that I don't think about my last conversation with my mother and her untimely passing.

The loss of my mother was a devastating reality. Her death illustrated the unexpected circumstances of life and the consequences of severe health complications. I learned a great deal about dialysis based on my mother's experience. Undergoing dialysis has numerous varying results: most are positive as dialysis performs the function of the kidney. However, it can take a toll on a patient's physicality or take their life during or after the procedure if too much fluid is taken off the body, which may cause one's blood pressure to drop and the patient to lose consciousness. The day my mother passed, I vowed that if I could help it, I would never go on dialysis.

Upon receiving my PKD diagnosis, I knew firsthand that I would have to take full responsibility if I wanted to beat this disease. My response required that I be fully engaged with my diagnosis, abreast of my medical options, proactive in getting proper care, and ready for the highs and lows of the journey I was about to face.

Chapter 2

MOVING FORWARD & ESTABLISHING HEALTHY ALTERNATIVES

To successfully embark on this journey, I recognized that I needed to establish a health regimen. The best plan of action I observed was how my mother approached her health. She implicitly complied with what the doctor prescribed while battling kidney disease. She asked few questions and did not waver as to why she should do anything differently than what the doctor asked of her. She was the model patient. She walked daily, used a nutritionist to guide her diet, consumed plenty of water, and got the proper amount of rest.

After learning that I also had the disease, I snapped to immediate action. The "in-network" hospital, based on my employer's medical plan, was good but not considered the best. I decided that I wanted to go to the best hospital. My wife jumped on this request quickly and began making calls leveraging her relationships. Upon talking to a colleague, she got me referred to a nephrologist (a doctor specializing in conditions that affect the kidney) at Johns Hopkins Hospital. Johns Hopkins Hospital consistently ranks among the top five hospitals in the country, so we knew we were in good hands. My wife and I believed it was important to have my procedure performed at a highly reputable research hospital as they would have the resources, experience, and knowledge to best extend my life.

During my first appointment, the nephrologist discussed PKD symptoms, causes, prevention, and complications with me. Afterward, I shared my family medical history. This education provided great insight into some of the challenges I might encounter and how we would try to address them. The nephrologist shared some different facts that resonated with me a little later.

- She said that life as I once knew it would be forever changed.
- She stated that studies concluded that PKD progresses quicker in men versus women.
- She suggested that I would be on medication for the rest of my life.

In shock, I sat there thinking, "What? But I'm in shape! I exercise! I run three times a week!" As I mentioned earlier, at that time, I had a group of men that I used to run with at SECU Stadium on the campus of the University of Maryland. For this reason, I was convinced that I could beat my high blood pressure history.

The last thing that the doctor said was that I might need a kidney transplant one day. Smugly, I looked at her, thinking, "Right. That's not going to happen, but I'll be sixty-five years old if it does. I'm a long way from sixty-five." Mentally, I was in a good place. I was stable, slept well at night, was not stressed, and was full of life. Little did I know what God had in store for me.

Next Steps

After my doctor's appointment at Johns Hopkins, I knew I had to begin doing things differently. Therefore, I established a regimen. My focus was to lower my blood pressure and get off blood pressure medication. First, I assessed what I was eating: I immediately went on a low-sodium diet, monitored the salt content in the foods I cooked, eliminated cooking, or placing salt on the meals I ate, decreased visits to fast-food restaurants, and began eating more fruits and vegetables. I never drank coffee, reduced drinking caffeinated beverages, and moved specifically to drinking water and sugarless juices. I learned the importance of staying hydrated regarding the kidneys, so consuming water became one of my top priorities.

Second, I established a weekly workout regimen. The regimen consisted of cardio (running three times per week) and lifting weights. In the winter, I would work out at the gym with a mix of running on the treadmill & riding an exercise bike. In addition, I would lift weights and do push-ups, sit-ups, crunches, and various other exercises to strengthen my body. As it got warmer, I went back to running the stadium stairs and hills once or twice a week and spent a couple of days per week on the treadmill. The stadium run was by far the best workout I endured. This training specifically strengthens your lower body by working your calves, quadriceps, glutes, and hips. In addition, it works your abdominal muscles. The intensity helps your cardiovascular system which, in turn, helps your conditioning and enables you to get in excellent shape. This workout really works all aspects of your body. However, the pounding going up and down the stairs would eventually take its toll—it was not good for my knees and, more importantly, my kidneys.

Third, I focused on getting the proper amount of rest and sleep. My goal was to get seven to eight hours of sleep per night. Before my diagnosis, I went to sleep late and rose early (it's no wonder I was tired much of the time). I learned that sleep is a critical component of a healthy lifestyle. If you sit down and talk to many executives, one of the keys to their success is getting the proper amount of rest each day and establishing a daily regimen. I bet most of them get seven to eight hours of sleep and exercise multiple times per week. Getting the proper amount of rest provides a lot of benefits:

1. Sleep reduces fatigue and helps you remain awake, alert, and at your best at all times.
2. Rest strengthens your heart: helps reduce stress levels, which can negatively impact how the heart functions and reduce high blood pressure.
3. Sleep supports a healthy immune system: which helps your body's ability to fight off viruses.
4. Rest reduces inflammation: poor sleep is linked to inflammation.

For these reasons alone, I am an advocate for getting the proper amount of sleep nightly. Getting adequate sleep will provide you with the energy you need to function properly. The best time for me to exercise is in the morning because I am refreshed, alert, and ready to begin my day.

Disciplining your body to rest as much as needed is a determining factor in recovery and rehabilitation, regardless of age. Our bodies function best when we establish a daily regimen—including going to sleep, waking up, and eating our meals around the same time each day. Though this process may appear boring to some, it is advantageous in providing us with everything we physically and mentally need. As a transplant patient, a daily routine is usually consistent with a healthy regimen; in doing so, we can be better prepared for upcoming procedures and speedier recoveries.

Bad News

Establishing healthy alternatives was a time-consuming process. I spent a lot of time researching my illness and how it impacts its victims while simultaneously trying to maintain my lifestyle and relationships. One day in the spring of 2006, I was at work and received a phone call that a college classmate and close friend had passed away. I was in a state of shock and deeply distressed upon receiving the news. The cause of death was a diabetic stroke. I learned he was feeling sick, went to the emergency room at a hospital, shared his symptoms, and tried to get a room (bed). Unfortunately, he was never administered to, nor able to get a room because the hospital was at capacity at the time; he died there while waiting for care. We probably will never receive the true story of what transpired, but the event was traumatic and very stressful.

The following day, I was at work and went to the restroom to use the toilet. When I began to urinate, I immediately noticed blood in my release—not just a little, but a lot of blood. I was speechless at first. After gaining my composure, I asked myself, "What is going on? This occurrence has never happened to me before. I need to go home immediately." When I got home, I called my primary care physician, and after several attempts, I finally reached him. I shared with him what transpired. I told him that I was under a lot of stress and about the recent fate of my friend. He asked how I was feeling physically, and I told him that I felt fine. Then he said, "This could be related to stress, but blood in your urine is a symptom of PKD. What probably transpired was some of the small cysts that surrounded your kidneys ruptured, and blood was released through your urine." The solution to the problem was to drink plenty of fluids, stay off my feet, and get plenty of rest.

Sharing the News

Given that episode, I called my boss. I decided to tell him what transpired and the details of my conversation with the doctor. To my surprise, he told me to get plenty of rest and stay home the rest of the week. It was March at the time, so he told me to watch March Madness, the NCAA men's basketball tournament, and follow my doctor's instructions. I was surprised by his response but seriously appreciated the empathy he shared towards me. He told me I could live with only one kidney as we talked. He shared that he had been injured in high school playing football, and his doctor removed one of his kidneys. He received the surgery and went on to live a very healthy life; the kidney removal restored him to a clean bill of health.

It is unlikely he would have shared his testimony with me if I had not opened up to him about my recent diagnosis. If he had not shared his testimony, I would have never realized he was living with one kidney. This situation furthered my belief that it is incredible how God uses people. That brief conversation meant so much to me because it illustrated empathy and that my boss cared for my health issues; he understood what I was going through and was willing to do what was best to get me back on my feet.

Ongoing Ailments

Throughout 2006 and 2007, I began to experience ailments and was completely dumbfounded about the source of these physical issues. As I said, I worked out regularly. There would be days when I would wake up after a workout and see inflammation in my lower extremities. My feet and ankles would swell, and I could not walk, or to walk, I would need crutches. I would think to myself, "Did I twist my foot while I was running? Did I land wrong while I was planting my foot? Was the distance too far? If so, why was the pain delayed if the injury was incurred the day before?"

Rather than see my primary care physician, I contacted a podiatrist (a medical specialist who helps address problems that affect your feet or legs) that I knew. The podiatrist shared there were multiple ways to treat the ailment. Upon having my PCP talk with the podiatrist, my PCP decided that medication should not be used in my treatment plan because of the adverse side effects it could have on my kidney. With this news in hand, I decided to put up with the pain and discomfort I was feeling.

A New Diagnosis

Unfortunately for me, the painful episodes with my feet and ankles started to occur more frequently. I learned over time that these bouts of pain I was experiencing were not injuries due to a fall that may have affected my ankle or foot but a condition called gout. Gout is a type of arthritis that is due to excess uric acid in the joints, which causes inflammation. This infirmity was extremely painful. The pain could last anywhere from a few days to weeks. It generally would start in my big toe and could expand to different areas of my foot. The attacks were significant, and the joints in my feet would become tender, red, and swell. I could not place any pressure or weight on my foot. The attacks would generally occur at night, and I would wake up in pain. I never knew what was happening until I was diagnosed with this condition.

Many people call gout "the old people's disease," as it is prevalent in men (and women) over fifty. Gout can be caused by excessive consumption of red meat (steak, beef, etc.) or seafood (shrimp, crabs & other shellfish), obesity, kidney disease, heart disease, and/or genetics. My medical team never mentioned that gout could be triggered through exercise. However, when I began to have trouble walking after a workout, I knew something was wrong. Some of the ways to prevent or treat gout are consistent with the regimen I established:

- Consume plenty of water and no beverages with sweetened additives
- Avoid or limit alcohol consumption
- Limit the consumption of red meat, seafood, and poultry
- Consume low-fat dairy products
- Maintain a healthy weight

Due to this diagnosis, I did my best to follow health-conscience guidelines and submit to my treatment plan—a process that was not perfect but proved to benefit me greatly.

Chapter 3

NEW BEGINNINGS

My gout diagnosis was the beginning of more significant changes in my life. In the summer of 2007, I received a call from my nephrologist. She said the medical team placed my name on the kidney transplant list. My nephrologist assured me that there was no need to be alarmed. I was placed on the list because my creatinine level dropped below a certain level. The creatinine test is performed to provide the doctor insight into a patient's kidney functionality levels. When someone's creatinine level falls to or below twenty, one is eligible to be placed on the kidney transplant list. This occurrence does not mean the numbers will continue to drop because they move around. However, the significance is that this process allowed me to begin accruing time on the kidney transplant list.

One November day before Thanksgiving, I received another call from my nephrologist. I remember that call like it was yesterday. I can tell you where I was located, who I was talking to and exactly what I was doing. In 2007, my employer, BearingPoint, hosted a leadership meeting at a major hotel in Washington, DC. While sitting in the conference's keynote session, my nephrologist called. She didn't go into much detail but quickly informed me she wanted to schedule an appointment for me in January. She told me to block off half a day for a series of appointments to meet with Johns Hopkins Comprehensive Transplant Center representatives. Once again, she emphasized that I should not worry; these specialists review transplant cases weekly and meet with patients to discuss their findings and make recommendations.

Another Announcement

In January 2008, my wife and I got some great news. We learned through another doctor's appointment that my wife was pregnant and that we would be expecting our first child. You can only imagine the thoughts going through our minds at the time. We were filled with joy and happiness and looking forward to expanding our family. We did not care if we had a boy or girl; all we wanted and prayed for was a healthy child.

Over the next few weeks, we were filled with excitement. As she did so well, my wife began planning for our new arrival. Naturally, we only shared the news with our parents because it was too early to start telling close friends and family. We began preparing for the baby by purchasing baby books, discussing the room our newborn would take, what room color we would select if our newborn were a boy or girl, the furniture we would need to purchase, and so much more. At this point, my upcoming doctor's appointment was an afterthought as we immersed ourselves in the preparation for our growing family.

A Not-so Routine Appointment

Meeting with the representatives from the transplant center was not a routine doctor's appointment; however, I did not expect any significant new findings to come out of the consultation. What I anticipated to be a regular appointment with a few doctors and specialists turned out to be much more than I ever imagined. The routine visit quickly turned into a half-day roller coaster ride based on all the emotions and thoughts going through my head.

That morning, I met with the transplant team, which consisted of my nephrologist, a nutritionist, a social worker, a nurse, a finance representative, and a donor coordinator. You name them; I met with them. The donor coordinator set the tone by sharing the agenda. The agenda included the purpose of the day, the people I would meet, and the roles each person played in how my process would move forward. Initially, I met with my nephrologist. She discussed the status of my labs. She also shared that she would continue to follow through with the recommended treatment of my illness. We discussed the transplants I might need in the future (these were consistent with our previous discussions) and my preference to never go on dialysis.

The nutritionist discussed the importance of my diet. She took it to another level by discussing the benefits of low sodium and a protein-heavy diet. She provided me with a list of recommended nutritionists I could work with to help me establish a diet that addressed my needs.

The social worker discussed my mental state, current job, and the type of support I needed pre and post-transplant. The finance representative shared all the costs associated with the surgery; the total could be upwards of four hundred thousand dollars. In addition to this expense, we discussed the monthly cost of medications post-transplant, which could be north of five thousand dollars per month. Lastly, we talked about Medicaid, which for transplant patients, covers eighty percent of the cost of the transplant. If I was asleep during any of the other presentations, by this time, they had my full attention.

After meeting with this team of medical professionals, I finally met with two young surgeons: one was African American, and the other was Asian. They stood out because they were young and minorities. I asked myself, "How long have these two young doctors been out of medical school and practicing medicine?" I remember that the African American doctor was from Louisiana and trained at the Mayo Clinic in Rochester, Minnesota. I don't recall where the Asian doctor got his training. However, I did know that these young men were some of the best at their craft, so I listened to them carefully.

Transplant Candidate

The African American surgeon asked me several questions. I do not recall many, but the one that stuck out in my mind was when he asked if I knew my blood type. I responded, "No," and asked, "Why?" Then he replied, "Well, we've been reviewing your case for a while, and based on what we see from your lab work, we believe that you're a good candidate for a kidney transplant."

Based on my lab work, they believed they had seen a trend in my numbers. They said that my kidney functionality would continue to decline and that they wanted to perform a pre-emptive kidney transplant. This diagnosis was consistent with what my nephrologist shared with me months earlier. He also said that they wanted to perform the procedure sooner rather than later because they did not want me to go on dialysis. Their rationale was that I was healthy, and the doctors did not want my health to decline further. If my health deteriorated and there was a negative impact on other organs, then there was a chance my transplant would have to be delayed, and dialysis would become my reality. Lastly, he shared that they could perform the transplant if I could secure a donor.

Reflection

After talking to the transplant team, to say that my eyes opened and my jaw dropped is an understatement. Naturally, my emotions took over at that point. I had a thousand and one questions with no concrete answers.

As I said previously, I learned my wife was pregnant with our first child just two weeks before this appointment. In addition, I began to question the financial viability of my company's operation. So, if I am honest, this new prognosis left me with more questions than answers. These were some of the questions going through my mind at the time:

- How do I go about getting this transplant?
- Will I get a kidney off the transplant list, or will it be a live donor?
- How long will it take to get a donor?
- Who will I ask to get tested to be a donor?
- Will I have a kidney transplant before my child is born?
- How can I provide for my unborn child?

And then the biggest question was: I've got a lot going on; where will I find the resources to pay for the transplant? Along with these questions, I was reminded that God, with His infinite wisdom, says, "I will provide!"

Statistics

The more I learned about kidney and liver diseases, the more I found out that I was only one in the vast majority of people afflicted by this disease. Polycystic Kidney Disease is a relatively common genetic disorder:

- PKD affects approximately six hundred thousand people in the United States and over twelve million people worldwide.
- It is the fourth leading cause of kidney failure and causes ten percent of all end-stage renal disease (ESRD), usually for people between the ages of forty and sixty. It can vary in how it affects men, women, and people of different races and ethnicities.

The more information I gained, the more I realized that I certainly was not the "only one" impacted by the disease. Additionally, I adopted the resolve to power through this situation, which had likewise affected many others. With this newfound acceptance, I decided to put one foot in front of the other and get to work. Now it was time for me to begin tackling my most considerable task: how to go about securing a donor.

Chapter 4

SECURING A DONOR

Securing a donor was a process that involved hard work, dedication, and resilience. I knew I had to establish a plan to help guarantee my transplant while juggling my other responsibilities. In particular, January 2008 was a month to remember: I learned that I had a newborn child on the way and needed to have a kidney transplant. During that time, excitement and uneasiness began as my search for a kidney donor began. The first few weeks after meeting with the transplant team had me paralyzed—I couldn't gather myself to move forward. It wasn't that I didn't know what I needed to do; instead, I was still in a state of shock that I needed a transplant.

The Approach

To help ease my concerns, I reached out to the two people I knew who had gone through this process before: my mother and a good friend. They each needed to identify donors to get kidneys but approached their journeys differently. In the end, they achieved the same result: identifying a donor. Similarly, an expression that comes to mind is, "there is more than one way to skin a cat." I considered several paths because there is more than one way to reach a destination. One is not better than the other; it just depends on the individual's desire to get to a specific goal.

My mother secured a kidney off the transplant list. Little did I know, my process of finding a donor began months before I even became aware I needed a transplant. My nephrologist referred me to get on the transplant list. I had been accruing time on the waiting list at Johns Hopkins Hospital for months (but this process could take years). I was aware that one in five people that need kidney transplants get them performed each year and that depending on one's "blood type," it could take even longer to find a donor. So, the quicker approach would be to establish a list of people I knew and ask them if they would go through the evaluation and testing process to become my donor. That is the approach my friend took.

After experiencing much trepidation, one of my closest friends said, "I will get tested to be your donor. Give me the telephone number of your donor coordinator, and I will get started." Naturally, the words he used were not that nice (he used a few choice words to get me off my behind). However, he knew what needed to be said and how the message needed to be delivered to get my process started. We can laugh at that conversation today, but it was no laughing matter in the winter of 2008. Nonetheless, I appreciated his motivation and frank honesty.

Family First, Friends Second

The conversation with my friend helped me jump-start my approach to identifying a live donor. I decided to develop categories of the people I was going to approach. I started by establishing a list:

- Family
- Friends
- Co-workers

- Wedding Party
- Fraternity Brothers

After developing this list, I began making phone calls. As noted, first, I started with my family and specifically reached out to my first cousins. Almost immediately, I eliminated my mother's side of the family. I realized there was a great chance those cousins would not be candidates to be donors because I believed they also had PKD (since it was hereditary on my maternal grandmother's side).

Next, I began reaching out to my father's side of the family. After making the first few calls, the cousins I reached out to started sharing their health challenges: high blood pressure, diabetes, kidney failure, and other ailments and diseases. While calling my family members and recognizing they weren't healthy enough to be donors, something dawned on me: my father came from a large family and was the youngest of twelve children. My sisters and I were the youngest grandchildren of Emma Lou and Jason Works. My first cousins were almost as old as my father and older than my mother. That led me to quickly conclude that most of my first cousins would not be good donor candidates because they were aging and already battling health challenges. My second and third cousins were much healthier, but I did not want to ask them to be donors because of their youth.

Alternatively, I began looking to my friends as possible donors. Outside of family, I believed that if anyone were going to become my donor, it would be a close friend—not a stranger. I knew that I would need to have a deep relationship with the people I would ask for them to agree to the donor terms. I also believed that the people I asked would need to be my age or slightly younger. If they were younger, there was a greater chance they had not begun experiencing the health challenges my older relatives were enduring. As I continued to develop my list, I inquired with my donor coordinator how I could approach the process more formally (not just by picking up the phone and placing a call).

Tailoring My Request

My donor coordinator shared that one of the best ways to approach potential donors was to send a letter or email stating:

- The kidney disease I was battling (PKD)
- An explanation of the disease
- My purpose and goal for the surgery (to live a normal life)
- The research that proves kidney disease is treatable with a transplant
- The necessity of identifying a qualified donor
- A request for their consideration in becoming a donor to address my need
- Encouragement for them to pray about this opportunity with a partner

This insight allowed me to tailor my request in a personal and inclusive way to the potential donor.

The Transplant Team

After my donor coordinator asked me to develop a list of potential donors, proceeding with the Johns Hopkins transplant team was a process. I remember being told that the coordinators would evaluate the donor prospects three at-a-time so that they could easily manage the screening process. First, the coordinator sent each potential donor a questionnaire to complete. Based on the responses from the questionnaire, the team determined if the candidate needed to proceed beyond the questionnaire. If so, they would screen them for infections and infectious diseases (because illnesses can be transmitted via transplantation). A candidate who tested positive for an infection would no longer be a donor candidate. Lastly, they began a series of tests to determine blood type. The medical team also took urine samples, EKG, radiological surveys, and many more tests. Throughout this process, candidates began to be eliminated from my potential donor list.

Once I was in tune with the process, I became very focused. Many people would ask me, "How did you approach getting donors?" I would reply, "Just like I was pursuing a deal at work." I approached the donor search process very methodically. In business, when you are *cold calling* a customer, it becomes a numbers game. For me to get five affirmative responses, I may have to call one hundred people. Naturally, some people will not answer the phone. Others will not respond to your messages, emails, or letters, and there may be some that will string you along. With the plan I developed, I intended to close in on a kidney donor like it was a sale. I stayed engaged with the potential donors. I knew when they were going to the doctor, insight into the results of their lab work, and their status as candidates. This knowledge was critical because as they eliminated individuals, I would ensure the donor coordinator was starting the process with the next person on our list.

Engaging the Support System

When engaging with a potential donor candidate, it is vital to communicate with the key decision-maker of their support group. Most times, becoming a donor is a decision that will not be made solely by the donor as there may be other people engaged in the process. That's why I asked each person that considered donating to pray about this opportunity and seek advice from their spouse, family, and loved ones.

If the candidate was married, I understood that the spouse would be involved in the final decision to donate because his or her action would impact their entire household. Given the seriousness of the request and operation, it was imperative to me that I include the potential donor's life partner in the decision-making process. For example, when I had a friend volunteer to get tested who did not first consult with their spouse, I declined his offer out of respect for his wife. I had no intention of causing strife in anyone's relationship based on my needs.

If the person was single, their parents or siblings might be involved. Once again, it could impact those not living in the household but close to the potential donor. A person could also be married but caring for their extended family (i.e., parents, siblings, nieces, nephews, as well as their own family)—a person with significant family responsibilities. That person may be healthy enough to donate but have too many things on his or her plate to be a viable donor candidate. There are numerous people and factors they need to consider as they decide whether they can be a donor or not.

Handling Rejection

With engaging a donor's support system, there is always the chance of loss and rejection. In pursuit of being good at my job, I also had to lose and be able to get back up when I got kicked down. And in case you were wondering how I managed rejection, I did so through the process of shock and humility.

One Sunday morning after church, as I was going through the process of securing a donor, I ran into the mother of a classmate from college. She pulled me aside and asked how the process was going to find a donor. I replied, "Well, people are getting screened and tested, but I have not found a qualifying donor yet." Then she asked, "Has anyone told you they would not get tested to be a donor?" I responded, "No." Then she asked, "How will you respond when someone rejects you?" Naturally, I said, "I don't know." Little did I know that God was preparing me for that first rejection. It didn't take long for me to hear the words, "I can't get tested."

That evening, I received a call from one of my close friends who said those exact words. I was stunned when he told me. I wasn't expecting to hear that from him. This friend and I were deeply connected, like brothers. I was also close to his wife, children, and parents. He was someone I could count on for everything (everything but a kidney, apparently). As he talked through his rationale, I understood why he could not proceed, but I was still in disbelief. I responded with humility. Fortunately, I was able to receive his decision, and it had no impact on our relationship.

Within the next six months, God clearly revealed why that friend could not proceed to get screened and tested. As I reflected, I was so glad he rejected me at that time. I learned that it's better to get a quick "No," than to have prolonged silence, indecision, or a "No," further down the screening process. If this friend had proceeded, been a kidney match, and had to decline due to unforeseen circumstances at the time, I would have been crushed. Trust me, I have seen that scenario play out, and it is not pretty. I accepted that God knew what was best for me. The experience taught me that although I do not always understand God's ways because they are not my own, I can always expect His way to be the best.

The other instances of rejection were not a direct "No." Instead, it was the absence of a response. On more than one occasion, I had friends and family share that they would get tested and then disappear. The actions spanned from excuses, unreturned phone calls, and unanswered emails. Additionally, some blamed others for their noncommitment (those not part of the decision-making process). I grew to be able to handle rejection, but I would have preferred that they be direct in their responses so that I could move on to the next person.

I learned during that process that sometimes, you must go with your gut. Suppose someone begins communicating with the donor coordinator and goes AWOL. In that case, they are slowing down the process for others who are content with proceeding. Therefore, organ recipients shouldn't allow the absence of others to stop them from executing their goal: securing a donor. And remember, obtaining a kidney is a *numbers game.* Time is of the essence. You can get over "NO," but you need decisions to move quickly versus lingering on.

Progress and Pitfalls

One thing that helped me through my journey is I had a prayer partner. As the process of finding a donor moved on, I prayed with him frequently. We prayed a couple of times a week and the focus had not changed. We prayed about a lot of things, to strengthen our relationships with our wives, draw nearer to God, cover our families, and gain favor on our jobs. We also prayed for the successful birth of my daughter and that I would soon secure a kidney donor. As the months passed, I began seeing God answer our prayers. By the summer's end, we identified one person that was a match to be a donor because he had the same blood type as me.

As I began getting closer to triumph, my breakthrough grew increasingly more difficult. On the health front, I was experiencing severe bouts of gout. The uric acid was building up in my joints and was becoming nearly unbearable. I talked to my PCP about treating it, and he recommended I try to manage the pain because medication might negatively impact my kidneys. So, my right hand swelled like a softball for approximately two months. As a result, I would go to meetings and shake customers' hands with my left hand (which is uncommon in business). Many times, I did not shake hands at all—I tried to hide my hand so I wouldn't draw attention to myself. Also, I had difficulty driving and placed the key in the car ignition with my left hand. I had to embrace doing things very awkwardly until I could have my surgery.

On the donor front, two additional candidates arose, and the doctors had not determined which candidate was the best to proceed with the transplant. They continued to run tests and saw some things that caused them to pause. It was not a question of *whether* they would continue but *who* of the potential candidates would be the likely donor (as things were very fluid). My family and I were very prayerful that the process would play itself out soon. We were also concerned about the timing of the transplant: would it occur just before my wife gave birth or after, as she was nearing the end of her pregnancy?

On the job front, things were also really heating up. We were amid the global financial crisis that began in 2007 and ran until 2009. My company was going through dire straits financially, and I was not sure we would stay in business. There were rumors that an executive group would see if they could make a play to purchase the company. However, when the financial markets dramatically declined (when Lehman Brothers filed for Chapter 11 Bankruptcy protection in September 2008), that option was no longer viable. At this point, I still had concerns about whether I would have a job when I eventually had my kidney transplant and the financial impact it would have on my family and me. This scenario was indeed the perfect storm.

Major Life Changes

In October 2008, my wife and I were blessed with our first child—a little girl we named Kylie Brynn Works. She was exactly what we prayed for: she had two arms, two legs, ten fingers, and was as healthy as she could be. She was our pride and joy and exactly what we needed to take our minds off my job and upcoming kidney transplant.

Just as we welcomed our new baby girl to the world, one of my three friends told me he was approved to become my donor. All the tests had gone through positively, and he had been screened for the kidney transplant. It looked like things were moving forward. My doctors had not given me the word yet, but I was excited that things were proceeding.

As I moved closer to my pending kidney transplant, I began to experience more difficult life changes. First, people were quietly leaving the company where I worked. No major announcements were being made, but key people were disappearing. People I had worked with for the past eight-plus years were being walked out the door. Leadership changes were taking place, and it was becoming clear what the long-term plan was for the company. Quietly, we could piece together that the company was being positioned to be sold. Fortunately, I was told that my position was safe and in a good place—at least for the short term.

Next, I began pressing the doctors to provide a date for my transplant. My donor was secured, but my company was going under, and I was adamant about having my transplant while I still had a job. Finally, we set a tentative date for January 2009, but it would have to be finalized over the coming weeks.

To complicate matters more, I injured myself at home a couple weeks after my daughter was born. I was getting out of bed when I planted my foot awkwardly one way and my knee the other. My knee was hurting, but I did not know the extent of the injury. I continued to walk on it for several days (as only I would do) until I could no longer place pressure on my leg. Upon visiting the doctor, I learned that I had torn my meniscus—yet another setback. I was given two options: have surgery or do rehab. Given that I would undergo a kidney transplant soon, I chose rehab.

For the next two months, I struggled. I drove to the rehab center three times a week, used crutches to walk, went to work, and tried to be the best husband and father I could be, given the circumstances. While this was not how I intended my first child to enter the world, this was our experience.

Making Strides

Over the next few weeks, things finally began to come together, considering all the setbacks. We locked in a date for the transplant, I completed rehab a few days after Christmas, and my family and I began getting ready for January 7th—the day of reckoning.

Overall, securing a donor came with many highs and lows. I never thought the career I chose and the training I received would prepare me for one of the most crucial sales jobs I had in my life: obtaining a kidney. The challenge of securing a donor to get a kidney and have a successful transplant was more important than any multi-million dollar deal I had ever closed. This sales pitch was about me living my everyday life and accomplishing my destiny. Given its significance and importance to my family and me, I approached it as such.

If you are ever in need of an organ donor, I want to encourage you to believe in your gifts and talents. You have to value your purpose. In business, I have always known that I am in the game to win when I am pursuing a deal. Even if three or four companies are at the table trying to win the business, I am always confident that I will be victorious.

God had already done a lot for me—so I knew He would not leave me now. My kidney was coming, and I was certain of that because of my resilient faith. I had seen Him open doors, put me in front of strangers, and bring me opportunities I had no business securing. By the grace of God, He had shown me the favor to win. Therefore, I believed that retrieving a kidney was child's play for Him.

All the steps it took to get me to this moment proved that securing a donor was a process that must be executed strategically. I learned quite a few lessons during my experience and will share them with you in the following chapters.

Chapter 5

THE KIDNEY TRANSPLANT STRATEGIC PLAN

D eveloping a plan to transform my health and overcome the challenges that could arise as a kidney recipient was key for me. To do this, I had to understand my challenges, the options for addressing these challenges, and the way to live moving forward. Although there is no cure for chronic kidney disease, there are ways to manage and treat the symptoms. One can manage or treat the disease through medication to address high blood pressure or cholesterol, but this will last only so long. I experienced this as my nephrologist monitored me for a few years. Over time, my condition worsened, and the doctor looked for other ways to treat me.

Treatment Options

Medical science can treat chronic kidney disease by placing the patient on dialysis; this was one of my alternatives. Dialysis is the process of removing waste products and extra fluid from your blood, and this process performs the functions your kidneys perform. The most common dialysis treatments are hemodialysis and peritoneal. Hemodialysis will require you to come to a dialysis center or hospital three times a week, four hours at a time, to have dialysis performed. The second option is peritoneal. This process is performed at home and generally at night while you are asleep. It also includes paying specific attention to washing your hands well, sanitizing, and taking the proper steps to connect to a dialysis machine. Next, you will have to connect dialysis fluid to a device that pumps the dialysis solution into your abdomen, filters your waste products, and cleanses your blood. This process generally takes anywhere from eight to ten hours per night. If you are considering dialysis, I recommend you consult your doctor to determine which approach is best for you.

Another form of treatment is to have a kidney transplant. This procedure will require major surgery in which you will have a kidney removed from your donor's body and inserted into your body. Some people must go on dialysis before having a kidney transplant. In contrast, others may have the ability to have a transplant before their kidney functionality declines to the level where they need to go on dialysis. After you have a transplant, it is imperative that you protect your kidney as though it were a newborn child. Many people have more than one kidney transplant—I am one of those persons.

I view my kidney as a gift from God that will allow me to live a normal life. Yes, I will have to be on medication and have my lab work done monthly, bi-monthly, or quarterly. Yes, I will have to endure countless doctor's appointments. However, I can live and function as I did primarily before my transplant, and those rewards are worth my challenges.

Game Plan

After I understood my treatment options, I developed a game plan on how to approach getting a kidney. First, I talked with my nephrologist and transplant coordinator. They provided options and guided me on the best route to take. One option was for me to get a kidney from a live donor or a cadaver (a deceased human body). The reasons I decided to identify a live donor included:

1. Shortened wait time: there was a possibility I could locate a donor whose blood type was compatible or a match and get a transplant within a year. Fortunately, this was my first experience; on average, it can take four to five years to get a kidney from the transplant waiting list.

2. Potentially optional dialysis: this was the case before my first kidney transplant. I credit my nephrologist for developing a plan for monitoring me and executing it to the extent that dialysis was unnecessary.

3. Immediate functionality: my transplanted kidney would start performing immediately after the surgery. Then, my doctor would want to see that my kidney was making urine as soon as possible and would observe and record my output accordingly. Sometimes that does not happen if a kidney is received from a deceased donor. In that case, my medical team would be responsible for waking my new kidney up to start functioning. There could be a slight delay, but it would eventually begin to work.

4. Longer useful life: a kidney from a live donor tends to have longer extended usage than a cadaver. This perspective was shared with me by my nephrologist, as well as transplant coordinators.

5. Allows the patient to plan and schedule the transplant with the doctors: I would get a call when a kidney became available from the transplant waiting list. The doctors would ask me to come for surgery at a moment's notice. I might get a call at 10:00 p.m. at night, and the transplant coordinator may ask me to go to the hospital immediately or at 6:00 a.m. for surgery at 9:00 a.m.

Either way, I would have to show up regardless of the inconvenient scheduling.

Proper Preparation

The next step in my strategic plan was to prepare my body for the transplant. First, I had to be tested and declared "determined to be healthy." A significant test that I had to take was a stress test. The doctors focused on whether my body could handle the stresses of a four-to-six-hour operation. For this process, I recall running on a treadmill. The purpose was to measure and monitor my heart rate and see how my body would respond to the running intensity. Fortunately for me, I have worked out for years, so running was not a challenge.

Furthermore, whenever I had a doctor's appointment after the doctor listened to my heart, they would generally ask, "Do you exercise? How frequently? Do you run? How long and how many miles do you run?" During these appointments, I was frequently told that my body functioned at levels younger than my age. This information did not surprise me as I depended on my exercise regimen to keep me young and in shape. My goal was to do all that I could to preserve my body.

Along with exercise, I worked hard to establish and maintain a healthy diet. My nephrologist recommended that I schedule an appointment with a nutritionist to help me establish a dietary plan. The nutritionist shared that I needed to begin preparing meals consisting of lean meats, fruits, vegetables, nuts, and grains. She also provided a list of food I should eat based on food type. It is no secret that people who practice good dietary habits heal quicker after surgery. Since my goal was to get back on my feet as soon as possible, my nutritionist recommended that I incorporate a diet consisting of the following:

- <u>Reduce protein intake</u>: purchase a kitchen scale and weigh the protein I consume daily.

- <u>Adopt a low-sodium diet</u>: reduce the consumption of foods at fast-food restaurants & heavily salted meals.
- <u>Find a salt intake alternative</u>: try garlic (or another vegetable) as a substitute for salt—it is a great way to add flavor to meals. Garlic is also a great source of vitamins B and C and protects against the common cold. Onions also represent an alternative to salt intake. This vegetable is high in Vitamin C, Manganese, and B Vitamins.
- <u>Shift to a low phosphorus diet</u>: consume beets, cooked carrots, corn on the cob, cabbage, cucumbers, lettuce, and potatoes (boiled or mashed, but soak them before you cook). Soaking the potatoes prior to cooking removes the starch and reduces the carbohydrate content. This is helpful with a low-carbohydrate diet.
- <u>Limit dairy products that are high in phosphorus</u>: consume them as directed by your nutritionist.
- <u>Adopt a diet that is low in potassium</u>: consume bagels, blueberries, strawberries, grapes, butter, and pasta, to name a few.
- <u>Consume vegetables that are high in nutrients</u>: vegetables such as cauliflower, cabbage, and broccoli aid a healthy heart, reduce cancer risk and provide an excellent fiber source. Cabbage is excellent as it provides fiber that keeps your digestive system healthy and allows you to have regular bowel movements. This vegetable is low in potassium, phosphorus, and sodium.
- <u>Consume fruits that provide high nutrients</u>: blueberries, strawberries, cherries (in moderation), and apples are fruits that contain various nutrients and are great sources of antioxidants for consumption. They are also an excellent source for protecting the body against cancer, heart disease, diabetes, and cognitive decline. Bulgur is a fiber high in Vitamin C, Manganese, and B vitamins.

Adopting a dietary plan caused me to focus on labels. This information provided great insight into the foods and ingredients I could or could not consume to establish and maintain a healthy diet.

Reaching Your Audience

Once I identified who my potential donor candidates would be and completed the proper planning of my physical needs, I decided to focus on engaging with my audience. I asked myself, "How will I reach the people I am targeting?" I didn't realize it at first but asking someone to donate their kidney to me was extremely difficult. Not every day a person asks another for an organ to be used for a transplant. I had to share with them that I was making this request because I was trying to live a normal life; this was a humbling appeal because I knew my life would change post-transplant.

To further illustrate this point, I relied on this Bible verse to soften my approach: "Greater love has no one than this: to lay down one's life for his friends" (John 15:13, NIV). This Scripture still brings me to tears because I'm honored that people considered helping me in my time of need. I was aware that a person could live a normal life with one kidney; still, it was a sacrifice not everyone would be able to make. So, I was all the more grateful for those who were willing to endure the process with me.

In the beginning, I contemplated many ways to approach disseminating my message for my needs. I knew that many people leveraged social media, which was not popular when I received my first transplant. Over the years, I learned I could place my request for a donor on Facebook, Instagram, LinkedIn, or any other social media platform.

For example, both of my sisters had kidney transplants. When one of my sisters asked my other sister and me to place a message on her behalf on Facebook, we happily obliged. She made this request because she didn't use social media. My other sister and I did, and this medium allowed us to post her message and reach thousands of people simultaneously. My sister received many responses—in some respects, more than we could handle. Social media allowed her message to be shared over other people's social networks. This "one to many" approach worked great as it got the message out and expanded our reach. The challenge with this approach is that the online environment is not controlled and can be difficult to manage. Therefore, we designed her message to provide details for potential donors to contact a donor coordinator at a specific hospital to start the process.

Another pitfall to seeking donors online is that sometimes there is no direct correspondence between the person posting the message and the reader. Due to the Health Information Portability & Accountability Act (HIPAA), the potential donor's specific health information is not shared with the person posting the message on behalf of the patient. Also, they may not be involved in the initial communication process or know the status of what is happening.

On the contrary, email was one of the main communication routes I used when seeking donors. I sent emails to potential donors and followed up with a phone call. This approach was personal, easy to manage, and was what I was accustomed to doing at my job. I approached potential candidates three at a time and followed up with them every step of the way. In addition, I learned when a potential donor was no longer viable—a trigger for me to send other candidates that were in line to continue through the process.

Some may not view this process as the best; however, it allowed me to be fully involved with my transplant plan. I was always aware of what was happening. It was important to me to facilitate the movement of the process. Furthermore, I can't say this enough if you are similarly struggling to secure a donor: you are your best health advocate. Remember that you are the one trying to obtain a kidney so you can have the ability to live a normal life. The sooner you identify a donor, the sooner you will have your transplant.

If you are still unsure about how you can get a kidney transplant, consider getting creative with your message. For instance, not too long ago I saw a man on the news who went to Disney World in Orlando, FL. While in the city, he developed a plan to have an informative shirt made. He wore the shirt to the theme park one day and requested those he deemed potential organ donors to view his online website. On the back of his shirt, it read, "In need of a kidney! Blood type is…call xxx-xxx-xxxx!" The shirt generated pictures taken by tourists, and eventually, his photo landed on Facebook. The man's story went viral with tens of thousands of shares, likes, and comments. Soon after, the man received a call from a man who was a perfect match. Let this man be an example that you must get your name and story out to the public to find your donor. Securing a kidney donor is no time to be shy. It is better to develop your game plan now to reap the benefits later.

Direct Donation

Another option I had to consider in my strategic plan was receiving a direct donation. In my eyes, this source is a blessing from God. I had to be on the transplant list to receive an organ via a direct donation. This distinction occurs when a person dies or is dying, and the family directs an organ for transplant purposes to a specific person. The process would allow me to jump to the top of the list no matter where I originally was on the transplant list. This process is significant as it can sometimes take a person upwards of five years to receive a kidney while waiting for a qualified participant.

Additionally, a direct donation is obtained through a cadaver. This door opens when a family recognizes that a loved one has been injured or is very ill and is not going to survive (based on the outlook presented to them by the doctors). Faced with this situation, the family will then decide whether they want or do not want to donate the organs of their loved one. At that point, the family will look to identify people who need an organ. The sick or injured person will likely be on life support as the medical facility keeps the organs functioning. Simultaneously, the family (and possibly friends) will identify potential candidates for the organs. Within a short time of the loved one's passing, the medical team will harvest the organs and transport them to the hospital, where the transplants will occur.

Finally, I am very fond of the "direct donation" process because I know firsthand its benefits. I know others who have been less fortunate because they were not on the transplant waiting list for one reason or another. Perhaps, when presented with the opportunity, they could not take advantage of it. Some members of my family have been engaged in this process multiple times before achieving success. As I share my plan, I want to reiterate how vital it is for donor recipients to explore all options presented to them to secure a kidney.

Getting My House in Order

I had to get my house in order to prepare for major surgery like a kidney transplant. This meant I had to generate a list of legal and financial documents in case my operation was unsuccessful and I did not survive.

While signing medical documents before my operation, I was asked two questions by the medical administrators. They were: "Do you have a Last Will and Testament," and "Do you have a Living Will (advance care directive)?" They also asked, "Do you want to be resuscitated or placed on life support if necessary for you to survive?" These were questions that I could not shy away from; furthermore, these discussions needed to also be had with my wife and parents. Given my daughter's ages as minors, these were not discussions I could have with my children.

In terms of documents, I had a last will and testament, living will, health care proxy, durable power of attorney, a medical history list, and so forth. Now, you may ask yourself, "How does he know these are necessities?" Well, my wife is a practicing attorney, so these procedures come second nature to her. I did not have to ask anyone else for legal advice following my surgery because I had her by my side.

On the financial end, I shared my bank accounts, investment accounts, 401(K) details, insurance policies, and other financial documents I deemed appropriate with my wife. As an organ recipient, I needed to ensure that my beneficiaries were also tied to all my accounts. Providing proper verification to access the family investments was (and still is) vitally important.

In addition, I ensured that all my billing statements were in order and accounted for, including my utilities, mortgage, insurance, cars, schooling, and more. Lastly, I gave my loved ones access to all my usernames and passwords. The purpose of this was to be prepared and not leave my family scrambling for answers if I passed away unexpectedly.

In summary, having your affairs in order in the event of a critical emergency is paramount, especially for organ recipients. These conversations may be challenging to have with loved ones and significant others, but they are necessary nonetheless (trust me, mine were with my wife). To be honest, I did not have all these conversations before my first transplant, but my wife began asking me these necessary questions before my second. My response at first was, "Do you think something may go wrong? Are you concerned I may not return to this house alive?" I eventually realized that although it made me feel uncomfortable, she was simply taking proper precautions. No one wants to have these conversations, but they must be had—the sooner they are had, the better-prepared one will be for a transplant.

Spiritual Foothold

Ultimately, it is crucial to recognize all components of a well-developed kidney transplant plan. This route will have sequential steps, detours, areas you may need to readdress, and tasks that are added along the way. Regardless, staying focused on the roadmap and being flexible with the results is more manageable when standing on a faith-based foothold.

To further illustrate my point, there are multiple evolving elements to getting a kidney transplant: spiritual, mental, physical, and financial. Some elements are consistent: everyday life, family, work, and other outside activities. These factors significantly increase the need to identify a transplant donor. As a result, I made sure that God was at the center of my roadmap. I understood from the beginning that this battle was not mine but the Lord's. To prepare myself, I started each day of my journey in prayer. I asked God to guide, encourage and lead my steps. Similarly, you will need a spiritual advocate to help manage all aspects of what is transpiring.

Please remember that in any position you take, you will have challenges. Some challenges will be so stifling that you may not be able to handle them collectively; instead, they must be segmented individually to manage. God stepped in for me during this time period.

Although my goal was to not let my challenges overwhelm my moments, God helped me with the highs and lows of my donor search. This process included disappointment from potential donors, delays due to health challenges, and even concerns about whether my body could consume the medication required post-transplant. He carried my burdens for me and removed them through prayer; He made my kidney transplant plan easier because He removed my "what if" fears. If you desire the same ease for transplant planning, I implore you to develop a relationship with the Lord so that He can help you strategize your best form of action. I guarantee it will be the best decision you've ever made.

Chapter 6

FACING THE FACTS (WORKPLACE PR STRATEGY)

N ow that we've covered the Kidney Transplant Strategic Plan, it is time to discuss another significant factor for organ recipients. Suppose you face a major operation and anticipate that your recovery time may hinder your ability to return to work (immediately or shortly after your surgery). In that case, you need to develop a workplace strategy. Your strategy will allow you to plan how you communicate with human resources, management, associates, and customers. Everyone you speak with will receive your news differently. Some people are very understanding, while others may not empathize with your situation. Therefore, you must create a plan to move your job forward and enhance the business in your absence.

The timing of your surgery and post-op recovery is generally never optimal, so disclosing this information will require your boss and coworkers to carry the workload during your absence. Being away from work for a few months can significantly burden your team. However, you can still accomplish this process through clear, direct communication with your colleagues.

Mentorship & Employer Communication

Identifying a person inside your organization who can or is willing to mentor you through the leave of absence process has many benefits. This is the route I took during my first kidney transplant, and my mentors served me very well. Can you think of anyone right now who meets this standard? Perhaps you have worked in an environment where you have witnessed a colleague take a short or long-term leave of absence from the job. This person may have been subject to a major operation or another emergency. Regardless of the reasoning for their time off, I encourage you to meet with this person to better understand what drove their decision to request a leave of absence. This colleague may give you a wealth of information and a pulse on how the company handles such discussions. If you are having trouble identifying who would be a good candidate, consider your boss, former boss, peer, team leader, HR. Anyone can qualify for this role as long as you feel comfortable seeking professional advice from them.

You can also gain further insight about medical leaves from someone external to your company—someone that has experienced communicating with their employer about taking a medical leave of absence. Learning from individuals who either work in or manage people in your role is very helpful. These conversations may also include how you will be compensated for time-sensitive business deals, and are essential to ensuring that you are treated fairly and evaluated properly. Ultimately, your job performance up to your leave of absence should be weighed by your superiors as they assess you against your goals and objectives—not by the time you will be away from work (which is out of your control). Your time away from work can be subjective, but you want it managed properly.

For instance, I worked in business development and sales after my transplant, so sales compensation was significant. During my absence and based on the closing dates scheduled, I knew that my team could complete a few of my business deals while I was on medical leave. Due to this possibility, I discussed with management how I could secure maximum revenue and compensation for all the deals I worked on—even in my absence. If the sale closed while I was on short-term medical leave, I had questions about being compensated for deals I completed. However, I could not find the answers in the company handbook or sales compensation plan regarding a short-term leave of absence. I later learned that management reviewed compensation on a case-by-case basis. In hindsight, I'm glad I raised these questions and concerns to ensure there were no issues upon my return.

At one point, I thought about strategically scheduling my surgery around deal closing dates. This strategy would enable me to be compensated for my sales if my company did not accept my proposed plan to get paid for closed deals. With words of wisdom, my father shared that if I delayed surgery to close a deal, I could get ill, which would significantly complicate matters. Then, I would deal with a much larger problem that could push surgery off for several months. Delaying surgery and becoming ill could have hurt me financially because I would have been forced to address medical expenses that could have been avoided. I could not risk furthering the health issues I already had in place. Therefore, I decided to take my father's advice and proceed with the surgery. As I look back on that moment, I'm grateful that he was able to mentor me through that situation.

In addition to finding a mentor, it is important to have conversations with your employer before going on medical leave. As I considered my options on how I would address requesting medical leave, I met with a friend who is an attorney handling employee benefits and compensation. I shared with him how my illness was physically affecting me. Fatigue was setting in, my energy levels were low, my attention to detail was waning, and I felt things slipping away and out of my control. My output was declining. As a result, my energy decline directly impacted my performance.

I knew I was going on medical leave at some point, but I was waiting for my doctor to give me the nod to proceed. My doctor responded, "You can approach this in two different ways: first, you can do nothing. You can believe that your employer will give you the benefit of the doubt. Maybe they will respond in a manner that supports you and your efforts to go on disability at the appropriate time. Or, you can take matters into your own hands and be proactive. Although your employer may already know about your health situation and challenges, you must protect yourself. You cannot expect management to evaluate you and give you the benefit of the doubt. You must make the optimal decision for you." My doctor said that if I was going out on medical leave, I could not leave the viability of my job in my employer's hands because they may make a decision that was not in my best interest. His interpretation seemed quite accurate, so I complied.

The same ideology is true for anyone in the workforce: employers will not be empathetic to a person's medical situation or make decisions that best support them. Depending on that person's elected health benefits, if they go on short or long-term disability, their employer is not responsible for paying them during their leave. Instead, they will get paid by the insurance company and Social Security Administration (SSA). Every pay period, social security is taken out of your paycheck. These benefits are yours, so no one is losing any money when this happens. This was some of the best advice I could have ever received from my lawyer friend. Knowing this information was vital in helping me establish an effective communications strategy.

When considering medical leave, it is also vital to understand the benefits package—the benefits that are available. To accomplish this goal, I went online to view the employee portal. Upon reviewing the information on the portal, I followed up by calling and emailing a representative in the human resources (HR) department. The HR staff provided sound advice on requesting and preparing for a leave of absence.

Then I explained the details surrounding my departure and included the estimated timeline. In response, HR provided insight into my possible options—short or long-term disability—and the best way to approach the process. I was grateful for HR's expertise because they gave me a better understanding of how my company operated.

All in all, the communication I received from my mentors and employers was priceless. With their shared wisdom, I made well-informed decisions regarding my medical leave of absence. If you are in a similar situation, I implore you to navigate these resources—I presume you won't regret this decision!

Corporate Culture

Additionally, understanding a company's corporate culture is critical when submitting a notice for a "leave of absence." A company's corporate culture represents its core beliefs, values, and standards of how it intends to operate. The corporate culture extends to the company's communication and interaction styles with its employees, company influences, ideologies, and how they treat their employees. The corporate culture is generally driven from the top down and preached by the company's CEO. Middle management must embrace the culture and how empathy is practiced. If they do not accept the culture, it will be difficult for it to resonate with the broader organization.

It is the company's responsibility to demonstrate its corporate culture to employees. For example, most businesses list these values on their websites. A company's publications will tell employees what is most important to the organization. Regarding health benefits, is your company one that shows empathy to employees with health adversities? Or do they embrace these challenges publicly and oppose them privately? I had to learn the answers to these questions to get a sense of how the leadership and middle management team would support or reject my situation. Therefore, I would highly suggest that all employees, particularly those with significant health challenges, gain the pulse of the corporate culture of their employer. Knowing this pulse will provide a sense of how an organization will respond to employees as they communicate their health situations.

The way a person's medical challenges will be received by their superiors is generally based on what they have been exposed to and experienced. For me, understanding how my employer handled medical absences in the past provided valuable insight into how my experience would be managed. Similarly, during your research, it is important to note the following:

1. Was senior management supportive of an employee's medical situation?
2. Was leadership understanding of performance changes due to illness?
3. Were there consequences for poor performance?
4. How was an employee received upon their return?
5. Was the employee expected to maintain the same workload or accounts upon return?

Responses to these questions will vary from person to person. However, thinking through them tells a person what they may be up against in terms of taking leave from a job.

I received great insight into my organization's corporate culture before my second kidney transplant. One day, I sought advice from a former boss on handling my health challenge. She told me who I should talk to in human resources when I should have this discussion, and how to confirm my medical options. My former boss told me how to share my transition with human resources and what length of time I may need to be away from work. She also informed me of my management team's anticipated reactions, how a leave of absence would impact me financially, and what she had observed in similar situations. She told me to remember that the company has a corporate culture, but departments and divisions have their own unique culture. How things are managed may differ from division to division, so it's best to stay current on the values and standards established by your company. As a result, I could better process and manage the corporate culture to my benefit.

Unknown to me, I had a colleague on my team battling an illness. I would have never known his physical state because we only saw one another twice a year. I did not know any details of his condition but later learned he was battling cancer. My coworker's situation allowed me to observe how our organization managed medical challenges within my division. Those team members who worked closely with him were very in tune with his medical challenges. As they carried the workload, my colleague's health declined. Unfortunately, his health deteriorated until he could no longer work. He was eventually placed in hospice care and passed away shortly after that.

What struck me was how the senior management handled the situation. As soon as he passed away, HR immediately filled his role. They appeared to show limited empathy regarding this employee's medical status. While my coworker was ill, some in leadership went as far as to push to fill his position (although he was still actively occupying it). What's more, I believe that management's lack of empathy could have negatively impacted his family. The company's approach was driven solely by a leader who desired full team coverage and maximized sales results regardless of who it affected.

Seeing the company's reaction up close, front and center, opened my eyes. Management's lack of empathy reassured me that I had to do what was best for me and that I needed to submit the paperwork to go on long-term disability. Doing so protected me financially and took the decision-making out of the hands of my employer; I would no longer have to worry about how my health may impact my employment. I observed how management handled my coworker's situation, so I adjusted my expectations accordingly. I learned that if I was ever in doubt about something, I should always put myself first—especially in the business world. Blindly trusting earthly leaders alone is a mistake because they are capable of failure. For this reason, I realized that I needed to place my faith in God solely.

Team Management

Once I developed a better appreciation for corporate culture, I had to figure out how I would prepare my coworkers for my absence. Therefore, I decided it would be best to give them a roadmap outlining how to proceed with working on the accounts I managed.

The first step in this process was to provide an understanding of the customer relations I had established. As a result, I developed a relationship overview that provided the name of each account, agency, or department, contact person, the status of the relationships (very positive, positive, neutral, negative, and very negative), deals, and estimated close dates. These details provided the team a framework for how they should proceed. It also allowed me to assign each relationship to a team member, which helped drive accountability. The relationship roadmap and an understanding of the deals gave the team the exact directions required to keep the deal pursuit process moving forward. Developing this map was a critical task because I wanted to ensure that the pursuit of the business continued to move forward as efficiently as possible during my absence.

Next, I provided the team with a matrix that outlined the deals scheduled to close in the pipeline over the next 90 days. This matrix showed each account, the contact person at the account, the status of the deals, the next steps, and estimated close dates. This matrix was critical as it also provided the regular cadence the team needed to use in discussing the deals with the customers. Also, it allowed our team to manage the timing of bringing on resources to start projects based on the estimated close dates.

Last, I worked closely with the senior managers and managing directors to ensure they could staff the roles for the engagements promptly. Our coordination was crucial to our ability to begin the projects quickly. Though there was a fair amount of back and forth, everything appeared seamless to the customer.

As new business opportunities became available, the team was prepared in my absence. We developed a plan to continue the deal pursuit process to position ourselves for future work. My medical leave was the first time I had been out of work for an extended period; however, our success was due to establishing strong teams and years of working closely with one another. Furthermore, I highly recommend that anyone going out on leave partner with their coworkers to ensure a successful transition of business productivity.

Unexpected Challenges

While partnering with my team to solidify future business deals, I uncovered a few unexpected challenges. In this subchapter, I will take a moment to discuss what happens when a employee goes out on disability. To clarify, an employer is not supposed to be communicating with an employee who is out on leave—that is standard procedure. My wife shared with my team that I had a successful operation, but no business discussions were ever had. During my first transplant, my boss respected this protocol. However, before my second transplant, my boss was not focused on the standards set by the company.

When I went out on long-term disability in June 2017, the business was going through a reorganization. The restructuring was not officially announced but would go into effect that July. When the reorganization was announced, I had been on disability for a month. By then, the reporting structure had changed, and my accounts had as well. My new boss was someone I knew and had worked for previously for six months. Within the first month of the reorganization, he called me, and we had a brief conversation. He shared some of the changes that would impact me, and I shared the status of my health. I knew I should have limited to no interaction with him while I was on disability, so I did not anticipate hearing from him. At the time of his call, I was laser-focused on my health and not thinking about anything work-related. Instead of calling to check on my well-being before receiving my transplant, he pursued a different approach.

My new boss called to ask me indirectly when I was returning. Then he started talking about job options and wanted me to consider accepting a severance package from the company. Well, this caught me off guard. First, while I knew companies offer severance packages during company restructuring, I did not know that would be offered to me—not because I had never considered it, but because I had always imagined the offer wouldn't occur for years down the road. Second, I had been on medical leave for five months and had not yet received my transplant. Considering these conditions, I asked myself, "Why is he discussing this with me? A *human resources representative* should initiate this information, not a *line manager*." Third, the insurance company was paying my disability benefits while I was on leave. As a result, it would've been their responsibility to forewarn me that my company was considering such an action. And fourth, my boss's approach was totally out of line.

I was aware that it was my company's policy when an employee was out on long-term disability, they must hold one's position for six months. After that time lapsed, they could advertise the position and hire someone else for the job. Knowledge of this protocol confirmed that my boss had no concern for my well-being but was focused solely on filling a slot on his team. When we spoke, I told him I did not have a kidney donor and there was no date for my transplant operation. In addition, I shared that after I received the transplant, it would take a minimum of 90 days for me to recover from the operation. This condition was contingent on whether I made a full recovery and was adequately healed from my surgery. His phone call screamed, NO EMPATHY! He did not care about me. His actions were manipulative and calculated, and I had a significant problem with his lack of understanding of my situation.

At that moment, I did not think about further addressing my boss's misconduct. I was more focused on my impending surgery and the recovery process to follow, so I chose to accept his callous behavior. In hindsight, if I had the opportunity to revisit this situation, I would have reported him to HR. His faulty managerial skills left a distasteful impression on me. My hope was that if this manager ever encountered a similar situation, he would respond more sympathetically to his employee than he did to me.

Likewise, when I later shared this story with a friend, he said, "Greg, don't take it personally. At the end of the day, when you're working in a large corporate environment, people are under pressure to perform. The only thing most people are focused on is the *bottom line*. So, you must stop worrying about *him* and focus on *yourself*." After reflecting on the matter, I accepted my friend's words of wisdom and tried my best to heed his advice. It wasn't long after this conversation that the words of my friend rang out as truth. Eventually, I secured a donor, received my kidney transplant, and recovered from the surgery (I will discuss these details more in the next chapter). When I returned to work, this boss was no longer employed by the company. I couldn't help but believe his absence was due to how he interacted with his team. Sometimes you reap what you sow.

Over time, I also had to consider that although I was getting compensated by the insurance company, it didn't cost my job anything to hold my position. The issue at hand was I was not generating revenue for the company—I could not provide value while I was away from work. Additionally, my boss's actions solidified what I had already learned to be true: the importance of reading an employer, understanding the corporate culture, and protecting myself. This situation further proved the value of understanding your company's business policies and the people you work with daily.

Career Moves

As mentioned, after my first transplant, I quickly transitioned back to work. The first step was to contact human resources to share my recovery progress and my return date. The HR representative suggested that I reach out to my boss to communicate my upcoming return, so I complied. Initially, I worked from home and went into the office when necessary. My team was very welcoming, and my boss allowed me to ease my way back into my work tasks.

Upon my return, I focused on closing the outstanding business deals I had set in place. I needed to complete those deals to secure my compensation. Little did I know that my company would file for Chapter 11 Bankruptcy on my second day back to work. At this point in our business world, everyone's lives were turned upside down: employees began scrambling to learn the status of their long-term employment. Three months later, many would find themselves unemployed.

The return to work after my second kidney transplant (more details to follow) was entirely different. This time, I was going back to work after a long-term absence. I had been away from the office for sixteen months. It was necessary that I confirm and coordinate my return to work with my medical team, the insurance company, and my employer. Normally, the process also required that my doctors clear my return to work based on my recovery. Then, I would communicate with the insurance company that I had been provided a return-to-work date. Once that was in place, I was responsible for communicating with my employer what that date was.

However, this return-to-work process was a bit different and was driven by the insurance company. The insurance company contacted me and shared that my disability was about to lapse. They had received word from my nephrologist that I was ready to return to work. The insurance company's goal was to be able to stop paying long-term disability as soon as possible. My nephrologist had cleared me to return to work, while my primary care physician had not. My PCP had not cleared me because there was a possibility I needed to have another procedure performed that was related to the kidney transplant.

Ultimately, there were details I needed to work through with my primary care physician and nephrologist before they could confirm their joint decision. These details required that I communicate with my doctors to determine if another procedure was necessary. While all this communication was happening, I was also communicating with my human resources team, keeping them abreast of what was transpiring.

Upon my return, the conditions at my workplace were different (as was to be expected). Given that I was in a revenue-generating job, I knew my position had been backfilled. I also knew I still had a job but needed to work with human resources to identify a new position. Human resources assigned me a specialist who worked with me to identify roles and set up interviews for jobs that I believed fit my skill set. If I did not find a job within 60 days, they would give me a severance package, and I would have to move on to another career.

Fortunately, I secured a new position in a different division within the allotted period. A new job still meant I had to transition slowly back into the workforce. It wasn't long before I was back on my feet and engaging customers in the workplace.

Documentation and Training

Throughout my experience facing the facts in the workplace, I've seen firsthand the value of documenting forms of communication among my colleagues and managers. The significance of this practice is for reference availability in the event of a dispute or misunderstanding. I encourage all readers to save texts, voicemails, and email conversations regarding any personal information discussed with management. Never allow promises to stand by word alone; you never know when you may need that information in writing to ensure your future job safety.

The ability to date a conversation, email, direct message, or text will provide you with factual evidence to leverage at any specific time. Furthermore, it will allow one to provide clarity around a subject and leave the guesswork out of discussions at hand. Proper documentation gives you all the information you need, readily accessible, to argue your point and diffuse any confusion.

In addition to documenting conversations, it is also beneficial for employees to embrace all training opportunities made available. I distinctly recall undergoing empathy training sessions focused on human resource effectiveness. During this process, my associates and I were given a book titled, Dare to Lead. The book's purpose was to discuss the importance of brave work, tough conversations, and whole hearts produced from job satisfaction. The experience was an eye-opener for me. It taught me how to approach employees with underlying issues and how to do so with compassion and understanding. The book provided me with a lens to see someone else's perspective, and I encourage others to read it for the same wealth of knowledge.

Salary vs. Hourly Wage Benefits

For those readers who do not work in a corporate setting, I understand that the disability process may look different to you. Suppose that you are an hourly wage earner versus a salaried employee. In that case, you will likely not receive full disability coverage. This advantage is usually reserved for full-time employees who receive a benefits package. Without full-time status, a donor-recipient would have to file for disability insurance.

Let me assure you that if you are not a full-time employee with coverage, do not be discouraged. As I mentioned before, my attorney friend was able to give me solid advice on my situation because he had undergone a similar medical leave experience. The law firm that employed him provided a benefits package responsible for covering his medical expenses. However, when he left the firm, he did his research and purchased health insurance options to ensure he had coverage to address any short-term or long-term needs he may encounter.

One blessing of being a kidney recipient is that Medicaid will pick up a percentage of the medical costs even without insurance. Medicaid will cover eighty percent of the costs of end-stage-renewal-failure (ESRF), a large part of kidney transplant expenses, including post-operative costs.

Whether you work for a business where you earn a salary or hourly wage, the same advice applies: take the proper steps when developing a workplace PR strategy. In summary, those steps include the following:

1. Find a mentor who can guide you through the process.
2. Communicate with leaders the circumstances regarding your absence.
3. Study corporate culture and effectively respond to business problems that may arise.
4. Manage your teammates and equip them with tools to make them successful during your absence.
5. Protect your role in the company by always practicing good business ethics.

These are the main steps I took to ensure a smooth transition during my medical leave of absence. As an employee of any type of business, being unable to work is never easy. However, I have learned along the way that developing a strategic plan is a great resource to aid you on your journey.

Chapter 7

A DAY IN THE LIFE OF A KIDNEY TRANSPLANT RECIPIENT

W e have discussed a lot in these last few chapters. Up until this point, you have learned what it takes to secure a donor, how to implement the Kidney Transplant Strategic Plan and ways you can utilize the Workplace Strategy to your advantage. As I mentioned before, I was eventually gifted a kidney not once but *twice*. The purpose of this chapter will be to discuss the details of those experiences.

At the end of December 2008, I returned to work after taking a few days off before the holidays. The end of the year was a bit stressful as I was trying to close the year-end business and prepare for the new calendar year. I knew that I would be on medical leave within two weeks for my transplant, so I ensured things were in order and provided a path for my colleagues to pick up where I left off. During that week, I received a phone call from my donor coordinator daily requesting that I come to Johns Hopkins Hospital to have tests run. I can't recall what the tests or exams were for, but I remember that the nature of the tests was fairly significant.

On the Friday before my transplant, one of the doctors asked if they could have me admitted one day before the operation. He wanted to ensure all the tests had been administered and that the results were positive. Being admitted a day early was a godsend for me, as I had been driving back and forth from the Washington Metro Area to Baltimore daily to run tests.I understood the importance of having all those tests administered, and I was willing to comply with the protocol. I knew that when surgeries are scheduled in advance, they must be performed on the day they are scheduled. It is costly to secure a room for surgery, and it would be a sunk cost to the hospital if the doctors had to reschedule because all the tests had not been administered. Therefore, I completed my work week and began to get prepared mentally over the weekend for my operation.

Support System

On Sunday, my family and I went to church. I had the opportunity to talk to many people there and pray with friends. I recall having a conversation with one of my long-time friends that got highly emotional. He asked me if I was scared to go under the knife. I responded, "No. If God had me wait ten years for my wife and me to bring a newborn baby into our house, I know the God I serve will keep me around to raise her." In other words, I knew my surgery would be successful.

Early Monday morning, my wife and I drove to the hospital for my transplant. We waited anxiously for me to be admitted and given a room upon arrival. Once I got into the room, I changed into the gown I had been given to wear. Then I was wheeled throughout the facility to the various testing locations within the hospital. There was no going back now.

After getting acclimated to my room, I started receiving emails—floods of emails coming back-to-back over my phone screen. The messages were prayers and well wishes from extended family and friends. All of this was happening the day before my operation. As I recall, I was overcome with emotion from all the love and support I was receiving.

Throughout the day, I talked to a select number of loved ones over the phone, but I did not see any visitors in person (which was to be expected). My mother laid the ground rules and stated that no one could visit me unless they were family. This decision helped reduce the number of people I had to entertain and protected my weak immune system.

In general, it is best for transplant organ recipients to limit the number of visitors that see them right after surgery to prevent exposure to germs that may cause illness. Surgeons have just operated and planted a foreign organ into the body, which is susceptible to rejection—following a kidney transplant, the immune system is truly at its weakest point. Furthermore, these guidelines are put in place to protect the organ and get you on the road to recovery. Outside of the medical providers, visitors are limited to reduce health complications, and you should comply with these regulations accordingly.

Likewise, my family enforced the visitation restrictions that were put in place, primarily by my mother. She wanted to protect me, and everyone in my support system complied. There were differences in my visitor list during my first and second transplants. During my first transplant, my donor and I had one outside visitor: a mutual friend who had supported both of us through this process. Our friend visited my donor first, came to my room second, and left shortly after. The only other guest my donor had was his wife.

During my second transplant, I must have forgotten the rules because I had visitors before my surgery and many non-family members afterward. At that time, I welcomed everyone that came to visit, and fortunately, I was not exposed to illnesses that my visitors may have been carrying. My advice to any transplant recipient, though, is to air on the side of caution if you are considering who can and cannot visit you in the hospital.

I would say that hospitals are much more restrictive of visitors for the modern-day kidney transplant recipient. The COVID pandemic has limited guests to one person: the recipient's spouse or significant other. In addition, your guest may only be able to stay for a maximum of twenty-four hours. Ultimately, having a strong support system that adheres to the medical guidelines laid before you makes a world of difference. All of this information is helpful to keep in mind when preparing for your inpatient stay.

Similarities and Differences of Kidney Transplants

In addition to visitation, there were several similarities and differences between my first and second kidney transplants. Little did I know I would approach these situations the same but receive very different outcomes. My approach to securing a kidney for my first transplant was to obtain a live donor. I asked several friends and family to consider getting tested and donating a kidney to me. After almost a year, I was able to identify and proceed with a live donor for my initial transplant.

However, for my second transplant, I received different results. I had countless people get tested to become donors; however, for nearly a year, I could not identify a viable candidate. Then, one Sunday afternoon, I received a call from one of my sisters. She said she knew a family who wanted to donate a kidney to me directly. I would learn shortly thereafter; this was called a direct donation. I was stunned by their generosity—mainly because a direct donation would allow me to jump to the top of the list for a transplant. As a result, I received my kidney from a family that had lost a loved one who was a registered organ donor.

Another differentiating factor between my two transplants is that I never had to go on dialysis as I approached my first transplant. My nephrologist was key to ensuring this did not happen and developed a plan accordingly. Her goal was to monitor me and proceed with a pre-emptive transplant only if her team determined my kidney functionality was declining and surgery was necessary. This proved to be the case, so after many people were tested, we were able to identify potential donors. From there, the doctors selected one out of three applicants based on who was the best match for my surgery.

While awaiting my second transplant, I went on dialysis. My nephrologist monitored me for years, but early on, she recognized I would be fortunate to get ten years out of my first transplanted kidney. Unfortunately, after experiencing biopsies, tissue scars, kidney functionality decline, and watching my body begin to dwindle, I was left with no choice but to pursue dialysis. Thankfully, I was fortunate enough to have my second transplant within six months of this treatment.

Another difference between my two surgeries was my recovery time. After my first transplant, I returned to work seven weeks post-transplant, but after my second transplant, I returned seven months post-transplant. Prior to being discharged from the hospital after my second transplant, the social worker asked me how quickly I returned to work after my first. Upon hearing my response, she shared that she believed I returned too quickly. Her guidance led me to better manage when I should resume my work duties.

Additionally, my decision to delay my return was also based on the swelling around my incision. My medical team had to pay careful attention to this area, and the drawn-out recovery time was not something I had foreseen. After some time, the swelling healed, and I was ready to get back to work.

In preparation for my surgeries, there was a difference in how I prepared for my departure. I believe it is vital to prepare for your hospital visits once you have a date for your transplant. I knew weeks in advance the date I would have my first transplant. This knowledge allowed me to pack my bags in advance and prepare for surgery. I packed a bag with my clothes, toiletries, laptop, phone, chargers, a few magazines to read, and my Bible.

Before my second transplant, I was not nearly as ready for surgery. Though I learned a couple of days prior that there was a potential direct donation available for me, I was in denial that it was really going to happen. In retrospect, I should have packed a bag as soon as I learned about this potential donation. However, I did not, so I was left scrambling when I received the call at 10:30 p.m. on a Tuesday night; the medical staff was requesting that I come to the hospital immediately for my operation. Considering this, I now know that proper preparation is key to reducing stress and anxiety, sometimes caused by surgery.

One of the main similarities between my surgeries was the doctors' post-transplant orders. After each transplant, my medical team encouraged me to get out of bed and walk. Their goal was to have me up, walking, and getting my blood flowing so that I could function once I was discharged. They did not want me or any other patient to be sedentary, lying in bed. Behavior such as this could have made me susceptible to blood clots. As such, I did what I was told. I walked around the floor at the hospital and wore compression socks to avoid the possibility of getting a blood clot.

Though I experienced highs and lows between both of my transplants, overall, I am grateful that God blessed me with two kidneys and two successful operations. You will learn more about my aftercare in the subsequent paragraphs.

Post-surgery

For my first transplant, my actual surgical procedure lasted between five to six hours. When I woke up, I realized I was in the Intensive Care Unit (ICU). Post-surgery, my donor and I were separated into different sections of the hospital by medical staff. One thing I would like to share regarding donors is that they treat them like royalty at Johns Hopkins Hospital. The hospital believes that given that these donors are providing the transplant recipient the gift of life, the least the medical staff can do is provide five-star service while they are recovering.

Overall, I had an excellent experience at John Hopkins as an organ recipient. After my first surgery, I remember hearing many things being said shortly after I woke up. One thing that stuck in my mind was a conversation I overheard about my blood pressure. I recall the doctors saying that they needed to get my blood pressure down. I'm not sure what my blood pressure numbers were then, but it was very concerning to my wife. I heard her discussing my recovery with the nurse when I looked over at her. At that point, I started smiling inside. I thought to myself, "I am going to be okay. They will get my blood pressure under control, and everything will be okay." I was grateful that I was awake and semi-conscious of my surroundings.

For the next twenty-four hours, I slept a lot. I had little to no desire to talk on the phone or see visitors in person. This response was considered standard until the anesthesia finally wore off. Once that happened, I experienced less pain. If I felt discomfort, I had the ability to press on one of the controls that administered pain medication. This option was beneficial. Before discharge, I was prescribed pain medication to take on an as-needed basis. While some people believe it is easy to become a painkiller addict, I quickly learned that I was not prescribed enough for that to become my experience—I have a high threshold for pain. As a result, I consumed only a few painkiller tablets once I was discharged from the hospital.

The first couple of days following both of my surgeries, I was primarily given ice chips to consume. Once I could process those without issues, the medical staff gave me Italian ice and soup. By the third day, I was primarily eating solid foods, soft foods (like grits) for breakfast, and mashed potatoes at dinner. Towards the end of my stay, the medical professionals removed all my dietary restrictions. With that said, the nutritionists highly recommended that I embrace a low-sodium diet. The focus was on managing my blood pressure while protecting my newfound kidney.

Additionally, after my surgery, my doctors were constantly checking me for urine and trying to measure the output. The medical team measured the output to observe that my kidneys were working correctly. Both doctors also wanted to check my creatinine levels (which are crucial to keeping the kidneys functional) to ensure that my numbers were going down until they stabilized. The monitoring of my vitals was yet another reason why I stayed in the hospital for the length that I did.

Recognizing My Blessing

I recall walking around the ward for the first time, the first or second day after my first transplant. I gingerly walked a couple laps around the ward. Initially, I was in pain, but I would take pain medications before walking. Over time, I slowly stopped consuming the pain medications. As I previously mentioned, my doctors and nurses would encourage me to walk multiple times a day. Each day I would walk a little further until I finally walked for ten minutes or more.

During this time, it was really helpful to hear and receive encouragement from my nurses: "Good job Mr. Works, you are doing great! Keep up the good work!" One day, after going on a lengthy walk around the ward, I returned to my room and broke down in tears. I knew I was improving because my nurses were supportive. However, as I began to walk by the other patient's rooms and saw that most of them were sitting or lying in their beds, something hit me.

I realized just how far God had brought me. I wasn't aware of when the other patients had their operations, their medical histories, or their expected recovery times, but I did know that I was fortunate to be in my situation. I knew that God had His hand on me and my life. I was walking around the ward twenty-four to forty-eight hours after my surgery, all while witnessing other patients suffering from their conditions. At that moment, I proclaimed, "God, whatever it is You want me to do, I will do. I will honor You. I will share my story with others. Whatever you want me to do, I'll do it." God had blessed me with more time on earth to enjoy my loved ones and fulfill my purpose. With the time I had left, I was dedicated to doing whatever it was He asked of me.

Similar to walking, there was another task I had to perform before I could be discharged from the hospital. Following my first surgery, I was required to do a simulation with the nurses. They role-played with me to ensure I could conduct household activities on my own or with little assistance. This event took place in a kitchen and laundry room. While there, the nurses asked me to demonstrate my ability to wash clothes, put up dishes, walk around, and function without someone's assistance. It was slightly comedic learning how to do these everyday tasks with my new kidney, but I embraced the opportunity. Naturally, I moved around gingerly because I still had stitches from the incision. However, by the time I was released, I was able to operate some tasks independently and was not a burden on my family.

When I reflect on the length of time for my recovery, I am still amazed by God's favor. The speed at which I healed from my surgeries was quick in my eyes. From a medical perspective, my doctors told me that my age and physical condition probably contributed to my ability to bounce back so quickly. However, from a spiritual perspective, I knew that it was the Lord's doing for me to recover as soon as I did. Receiving and healing from my kidney transplant was indeed a humbling experience.

Non-negotiables

My doctors started me on medications immediately after my transplant. Some of the prescriptions included anti-rejection meds, blood pressure meds, and one pill (I cannot recall the name of) that was so big that I struggled to swallow it. Following these medications, I quickly learned that there were several non-negotiables involved in post-surgery—taking my meds was one of them. The nurses were sure to remind me that regardless of how I felt, the one thing that I could not do post-op was skip my medications. I had to take my medicines as they were prescribed.

The doctors initially told me to take my medication four times a day: 8:00 a.m., 10:00 a.m., 2:00 p.m., and 8:00 p.m. They taught me the importance of taking my medication on time and told me to use the alarm on my cell phone if I needed a reminder. Naturally, when I was in the hospital, the nurses gave me my medication, but once I was released, I embraced the practice of consuming my medicine on my own. The pharmacists provided a pill case so that I could segment the medications I took by day and time. I knew how important it was not to skip my prescriptions because I was not allowed to double the dose. Skipping my allotted time for meds could have severe consequences, and I was not willing to risk it.

It is important to note that organ recipients will take medication for the rest of their lives. Some will be prescription drugs, while others may be over-the-counter. Over time, the doctors will wean you off some as they were prescribed to be taken for a certain period after the transplant. Regardless of what the recommendation is, the medicines you are given will be used to address a specific condition. And rest assured, your doctors will monitor your progress based on in-person appointments, blood work, labs, and other tests that may be needed.

I am reminded of an analogy a kidney transplant friend once shared with me. He said that being a kidney transplant patient is unique because it's like making chili: the doctors will mix all kinds of ingredients and make changes until they get the numbers right. Once the numbers are stable, the doctors will move forward and continue to monitor the blood work for bodily changes.

Last but not least I can say that monitoring one's vitals is yet another non-negotiable for post-op patients. To this day, I am required to check my temperature, blood pressure, pulse, and weight daily for sudden changes. While doing these activities may seem tedious, the process lets me know where I stand health-wise.

In summary, a day in the life of a kidney transplant recipient can vary from person to person. My experience was primarily positive due to the excellent services provided by John Hopkins Hospital, the caring medical staff, my supportive family and friends, and my loving God, who secured me throughout it all. All these factors contributed to a restful post-operation and promising recovery.

Chapter 8

RECOVERY

D uring the recovery process post-operation, organ recipients should continue taking their medications as prescribed and develop a regular exercise plan. This action plan will allow them to reduce or manage weight gain, blood pressure, cholesterol levels, stress levels and potentially increase energy.

Further instructions include avoiding lifting anything heavier than ten pounds up to four weeks post-transplant. Organ recipients should avoid doing sit-ups for the first six months. They should avoid this exercise because the incision from surgery is around their abdomen, and there are stitches where the kidneys are sewn. Doctors don't want recipients lifting anything heavy that could separate the stitches or cause a hernia. Part of the recipient's recovery will also include eating healthy, balanced meals and avoiding foods high in sugars and fat. Ultimately, recipients that submit to these practices are more likely to have a faster recovery.

Rest

To further accelerate my recovery, one of the most important things I did post-transplant was to stay at home. My focus was on healing as quickly as possible because my immune system was at its weakest immediately after my transplant. So, I didn't want to expose myself to germs or anything else that could attack my health. Sleep was paramount post-transplant, as I was not sleeping through the night prior to my operation. During those first few months, I did not welcome visitors into my house to protect myself (given that I had a compromised immune system). My wife placed masks and hand sanitizer at the door in the event we had guests as an added layer of safety.

In addition, I always wore a mask when I traveled to doctor's appointments to get my labs (initially, they were twice a week). My doctors also shared that I should not drive while still on pain medication until my stitches were removed. My steps represented protective measures for the first six weeks after my surgery.

My support system truly served my family and me during this time. Initially, my mother-in-law came from out of town to help transport me to doctor's appointments. After her departure, my wife, parents, and friends transported me. Outside of doctor's visits, I spent as much time as possible resting and sleeping at home. Spending the majority of my time recovering at home was one of the best decisions I could have made post-surgery. I always encourage others in similar situations to do the same.

Returning to Everyday Activities

My medical team cleared me to return to work six weeks after my first transplant. By now, a few changes had transpired, including:

1. I was off pain medications
2. My stitches had been removed
3. I returned to driving

These improvements made me anxious to return to work and resume my regular duties. At first, I worked virtually from home, but I was finally back in the office roughly two months after my surgery.

You would never know how I was feeling based on my appearance. Things looked great externally, but internally, I was having challenges with my first kidney. Within the first twelve months of surgery, my lab reports detected signs of rejection. Unfortunately, I could not consume a complete dosage of one of the anti-rejection medications. When the doctor prescribed a larger dose, my body could not consume it, and as a result, it caused scarring of the kidney tissue. I learned a few years later that the reduced dosage impacted the functionality of my kidney; this was a significant reason I experienced signs of rejection.

As a result, the average life of my first transplanted kidney was reduced. The goal of this transplant was to treat my kidney disease and allow me to continue experiencing everyday life. It served its purpose for several years, and the signs of rejection did not initially impact my daily activities. However, eventually, the doctors recognized the average life of this kidney was declining. I did everything I could to protect my kidney: ate right, hydrated, exercised regularly, and took my medications. None-theless, my body responded adversely, which eventually led me to need a second transplant.

After securing another donor (I'll discuss this experience in detail later), my second transplant was performed on Valentine's Day, February 14th, 2018. *What a gift!* Upon discharge from the hospital, I spoke to the social workers about a return-to-work date. They shared that I should take my time to experience a full recovery and to "Listen to my body." They also shared that they had seen some patients delay their return to work for almost a year. At one of my follow up appointments, the doctor noticed I had swelling around my incision. The belief was I may have experienced a hernia which would cause me to have another operation. Rather than recommend that I return to work quickly, the medical staff monitored the potential hernia. In mid-September 2018, I was finally cleared to return to the office.

Protecting My Gift

My transition was coming together slowly but surely as I bridged the gap between the three R's: recovering, returning to work, and renewing my health. I was grateful for this progress because it confirmed that my health was headed in the right direction as I reembarked on my work journey. In addition to protecting myself from unwanted germs, it was important to me to defend myself from actions that may cause kidney damage.

For example, most doctors recommend that all post-transplant patients refrain from smoking. Therefore, I do not engage with tobacco in any way. Smoking can cause damage to vital organs and can result in cancer. Post-transplant patients should also avoid drinking caffeinated beverages such as soft drinks and coffee. In addition, it is best to avoid being in crowded environments with high exposure to germs until the immune system is strong enough to protect itself. As a result, I fully embrace social distancing.

During the COVID pandemic especially, I encourage all readers to take the proper precautions in public: wear your mask, stay socially distant, and get vaccinated and boosted because organ recipients are especially susceptible to illness. Many transplant patients' post-vaccination did not have antibodies to protect themselves against COVID and its variants. As such, after doing some research, I learned that many transplant patients who had two vaccination shots and multiple booster shots still came down with COVID. Therefore, it is crucial to guard yourself against germs if you are an organ recipient.

Some organ recipients have experienced extended hospital stays and even fatalities due to virus exposure. For example, one of my friends received a kidney and liver transplant in the winter of 2021. I ran into him a few months after his transplant at a cookout. I noticed that he was surrounded by people and was not wearing a mask. He did not have a valid rebuttal when I expressed my disappointment with his current decisions. I told him, "Out of all people and after everything you've gone through, you need to take better care of yourself. You are your best health advocate. No one must want you to be healthy more than yourself (and, likely, your spouse). You must do what's right for your body, even if that means making difficult or unpopular decisions."

After having that conversation, it became clear to me that not all doctors are the same, nor do they provide the same care and advice for their patients. My friend was either unaware that he was supposed to be socially distanced following his operation or was ignoring his doctor's recommendation. Kidney transplant recipients cannot operate as people without this illness do—they need to be overly cautious in all settings. For instance, I was at a medical facility for five minutes, having my labs drawn, and was exposed to this lethal virus. I learned then that it does not take much to get exposed to sickness. My COVID experience showed me that my friend and probably many other donor recipients operate recklessly or out of ignorance or defiance. In return, their carelessness threatens those who actively practice proper precautions against the virus.

With this scenario in mind, I understood that donor recipients must educate themselves on what they should or should not be doing. As for me, even when taking the "right steps" to keep my organ safe, I still experienced some fearsome challenges and setbacks. Nonetheless, I believe that protecting my kidney—the best way I know how—is key to enduring a successful new organ experience.

Support System Post-surgery

After my transplants, I socially isolated myself from my family. I put this behavior into practice to protect myself because of my weak immune system. As "super supporters," my wife and mother-in-law brought me food, beverages, and other essentials throughout the day. Meanwhile, I caught up on my sleep, aiming for eight hours of rest daily. Their constant support helped accelerate my recovery.

After my first kidney transplant, I spent most of my time in the basement watching TV, reading, and resting. I specifically remember watching the 2009 presidential inauguration honoring Barack Obama during that time. As I watched the celebration from my basement, I felt encouraged; it was a monumental moment in United States history. I was grateful that my support system granted me the opportunity to enjoy the inauguration from the comfort of my home.

In addition, the rest of my family and friends tremendously impacted how quickly I got back on my feet. Many of our loved ones reached out after my surgery and provided meals for my family and me. My wife's sorority sisters and other members of the organizations she participated in sent us gift cards to purchase meals from restaurants (we tried to focus on low-sodium businesses). My classmates from Howard University pooled their resources to get a classmate (and friend who is a caterer) to prepare meals for my family.

At one point, we had accumulated so much donated food that we had to invest in a small freezer to store the meals and leftovers. That needed purchase was a great problem to have! We incredibly appreciated this giving because such generosity took a lot of pressure off my wife.

Throughout both surgeries, I felt love from my family, friends, co-workers, and peers; I was lacking for nothing. The experience taught me that it takes a village to recover from receiving an organ and that I could not have recovered as quickly without all the hands that supported me.

Showing Gratitude

Throughout the process, you must show gratitude to those you have engaged with during the transplant process. First, I expressed my appreciation to all the people who considered being my donor. I recognized some people responded quickly, slowly, or delayed, while others never responded. Yet, I respected their decisions regardless of the responses or lack thereof they gave. My duty was to accept whatever communication I received and thank them for their consideration.

Second, I appreciated all the medical staff that helped me along the way, including the nurses, social workers, financial consultants, doctors, and surgeons. Each played a vital role in my recovery and served me throughout both recipient processes.

Third, it was vital for me to send "thank you" notes to all the people that provided me and my family meals while I was recovering. Taking that burden off my wife as she was trying to support me, manage our house, and keep up her workload, was a great aid to our family.

Lastly, I thanked my relatives who were there for me at the hospital and visited me post-transplant. They took me to doctor's appointments and filled the voids when my wife could not assist. Since I experienced two transplants in my lifetime, I wanted my family to know how much I appreciated them for supporting me in my times of need. If I may need another transplant (though I pray that is not the case), I hope that everyone involved during my first two will feel called to support me again.

Allying with My Doctor

In hindsight, I believe I experienced a speedy recovery because I had a great support system and submitted to the doctor's orders. In addition, based on my relationship with God, I knew He would place the right medical practitioners in my life to lead me to a successful recovery.

Similarly, I encourage readers recovering from a kidney transplant to heed the advice of their medical practitioners. I was always transparent with my doctors about how I felt and wanted them to address my medical needs and concerns. Also, I listened quickly to their recommendations because they had experience working with hundreds of patients and were the experts. I rarely wavered from the doctor's orders unless I heard God telling me not to adhere to them, and I would encourage everyone else to do the same.

Organ recipients should also listen to their bodies and report adverse reactions to medications to their medical team. I followed this advice and eventually questioned some of my prescriptions. Upon further analysis from my doctors, they offered medicines that were better for me. This example demonstrates that there is give and take involved in your recovery process. However, ultimately, it is the recipient's job to follow the directions of their medical providers.

Chapter 9

TRANSFORMATION

Following my transplants and recoveries throughout my life, I have experienced a great transformation. When I look at all the events that have occurred, I understand that they touch my mind, body, and soul:

1. October 2008, my first daughter was born
2. January 2009, I underwent my first kidney transplant
3. February 2009, my employer filed for Chapter 11 bankruptcy
4. May 2009, I lost my job
5. August 2009, I started a new job
6. January 2010, my second daughter was born
7. January 2013, my mother passed away
8. February 2018, I underwent my second kidney transplant

To reiterate, these events took place over ten years and proved to me that I was not guaranteed the vigorous health of my youth. As a kidney recipient, I quickly learned that I would be medically monitored for the rest of my life. Moreover, I would have doctor's appointments every four months to monitor my kidney. Those observations would extend to bi-annually over time; I would be required to take medication daily; I would go to the hospital or laboratory facility monthly and submit blood work for labs. Eventually, based on those labs, my doctors identified a trend that my kidney functionality was declining—which led to my second transplant.

In between my transplants, as my kidney functionally began to decline, the symptoms of end-stage renal failure (ESRF) became very apparent. Five to six years after my initial transplant, I began to experience symptoms of anemia such as fatigue, dizziness, and cold hands and feet. I experienced physical ailments such as sleeping problems, frequent urination, and fluid retention, to name a few. Then one day, a little less than six years from the date of my initial transplant, my nephrologist shared that I would need a kidney for a second transplant at some point down the road.

Alarming Symptoms

A few years after my first transplant, I endured an alarming incident. I was working in my home office when suddenly, I caught myself beginning to doze off. When this began to happen more frequently—mostly at night but sometimes during the middle of the day—I grew more concerned. I felt like I was fading fast and would not be able to maintain the pace needed to excel in my workplace. Considering that I was growing older, I knew that I could not push myself past my limits anymore.

It was long after I made this determination that I later learned that fatigue was a significant symptom of ESRF. ESRF was the reason I was fading during the day and dozing off to sleep. After running some tests, my doctors concluded that my hemoglobin levels were declining. My red blood cell count was also low, which was a by-product of kidney disease. To address the fatigue and increase my red blood cell count, the doctor requested I visit the medical office bi-weekly to get an Epogen shot. The benefit of this shot was to increase my red blood cell count and provide me energy to continue performing my daily activities.

Another symptom of ESRF was frequent urination, another symptom of mine at the time. I started tracking how frequently I needed to go to the bathroom. So, I would monitor the output of urine produced so that I could share it with my doctors. It was strange that my urine output did not seem to match the urge or need to urinate, but that was the case. Naturally, the result was a decrease in my weight. These symptoms were signs that my new kidney would not last forever.

Indeed, my kidney was never guaranteed to last a lifetime, even if I had taken perfect care of myself. Within the first twelve months of my initial transplant, I had a biopsy on my kidney. At this appointment, my nephrologist recognized some underlying issues: I had experienced tissue scarring on and around my transplanted kidney. I was also unable to consume a full dose of the anti-rejection medication, making it difficult for the kidney to be fully protected. These were hiccups that would need to be addressed sooner rather than later.

The goal of my nephrologist was to monitor my kidney and prescribe the proper medications to protect it. The average useful life of a transplanted organ from a live donor was ten-plus years, which was also my medical team's target. Fortunately for me, I made it to nine years. I always knew the risks of inserting a foreign organ inside my body because my immune system might attack the transplanted kidney. Hence, I was always susceptible to rejection.

In hindsight, I am grateful that I received a direct donation for my second kidney and that it was a successful operation. My prayer is that my current kidney will last longer than my first and that my children will never have to experience kidney failure.

Work-life Balance and Future Career Goals

After my transplants, not only did I transform physically, but the way I approached my career responsibilities transformed as well. In the workplace, one of the concepts most people strive for is work-life balance:

balancing the time spent working against the time spent with friends and family and doing other activities that one enjoys. Unfortunately, I have never worked in an environment with a work-life balance—my experience has been quite the contrary. I have always worked in very stressful environments, quickly logging sixty-plus hours a week before my first kidney transplant. Almost immediately after my diagnosis, I recognized that moving forward, it didn't make sense for me to return to that work environment.

As I mentioned before, I was in a unique situation because I went back to work seven weeks after my first kidney transplant. A day after I returned, my firm filed for Chapter 11 bankruptcy protection, and three months later, I was out of a job. Naturally, I was anxious, but most importantly, I had already received my first kidney transplant and was now in need of new employment.

Fortunately, my job search provided several options for employment. Recruiters presented me with four to five different opportunities that varied from role to role, and I received multiple job offers based on my interviews. As I examined my options, I looked at less demanding jobs similar to my old position.

Upon accepting my first job post-transplant, I returned to a previous employer. I made this decision because I knew I could excel quickly there due to my familiarity with the role, staff members, and customers. This would also reduce the learning curve and enable me to add immediate value to my new team.

I was also stepping into my new role as a father at the time. I knew it would not be smart to take on the same stress level in my new role that I had in my old role. I also realized that what I deemed important pre-transplant was no longer the same. Trying to *earn the gold watch* and *climb the corporate ladder* was no longer the main priority in my life. I was a family man and recovering kidney recipient now, so I had to make decisions accordingly.

As I reflect, I am satisfied with my postoperative career decisions. I wanted to be as fully invested in my family's life as possible, and I needed a career that would give me the flexibility to do so. Therefore, I focused on finding a new job opportunity that gave me peace of mind. I also required an attractive compensation package to help cover the cost of my bills and save for my children's education and my retirement. God allowed career goals to fall into place according to His will, with my family at my side. I will forever be grateful for His covering.

Family First

From the time I learned I needed a kidney until the birth of my two daughters, I have transformed how I treat my loved ones. Becoming a father made me appreciate the importance of living a healthy lifestyle and establishing a legacy. I would not be able to impact future generations if my family was not one of my top priorities. I wanted my children to reflect on their youth and be proud of the father I was to them. A supportive father who attended all their events, helped with their homework, and provided sound advice in their times of need.

I especially wanted to be available to my wife and sensitive to her needs as my spouse. For example, in January 2010, my job hosted a national sales meeting in Dallas, TX. At the time, my wife was days away from delivering our second child. The timing of this meeting couldn't have been worse. I knew I was obligated to attend this meeting, but I also knew I needed to be close to home if my wife went into labor.

I remember approaching my boss with this dilemma and wondering how he would respond. I said, "I can't attend the sales meeting this year. My wife is expecting, and our child could come any day now." His response was surprisingly supportive. If I had not shared this issue with him and requested to remain in the office rather than attend that sales meeting, I could have potentially missed my daughter's birth. If that happened, it would've been very difficult for me to forgive myself. This situation is another example of why it is important to keep family first.

By the same token, my post-operation mindset taught me that I never wanted to miss opportunities to spend time with my children. I wanted to be in town to attend their school functions if my work travel schedule permitted. If I was in a meeting, I wanted to be able to leave early. If I had to take a phone call, I wanted the option to take the call during my commute time. I desired to be the type of father who would sacrifice his work schedule for his family, and I hold this same concept true today.

If you are a future donor recipient, I want you to remember that your family should be a part of your transformative journey. Your family should learn to adapt to the new you as you recover. As a team, all parties can experience growth as they find balance in your new life stage.

Faith Increase

Another segment of transformation that I experienced post-surgery was the increase in my faith. I was already a person who walked in faith and followed God. Specifically, I had taken Bible Institute and discipleship classes and ministered to men for years. I had been very active and served on the Men's Ministry Leadership team at my church. And most importantly, I had been building a relationship with God since my youth. However, the reality of my surgery took my spiritual beliefs to another level. Seeing how God protected me, brought donors to me, and healed me proved how only God could orchestrate those transformative events.

First, I was humbled by the number of people who considered being my donors and getting tested. Second, most of my candidates kept me abreast of their progress and made me aware of whether they could or could not proceed as donor candidates. Their transparency was vital because it kept the process going. Third, as donor candidates were going through the testing process, I recognized that God had His hand on me every step of the way.

I was constantly reminded that God showed me favor. God kept my position secure while my wife was pregnant with our first child amidst chaos and layoffs. He covered me while I was on short-term disability, recovering from surgery. In addition, it was no coincidence that my company filed for Chapter 11 on the second day after my return and that I was able to find a replacement job shortly after. It's as if God told me, "Don't worry, I got you." God's mercy and grace over my circumstances propelled my faith and caused me to experience significant spiritual growth.

When I look at how I received the kidney for my second transplant, I am astonished by God's ways and timing. I had been on the transplant list for almost eighteen months, aggressively seeking a kidney for over a year. One week, I had no potential donors, and the following week, I received a call with a direct kidney donation that came out of nowhere.

God had been orchestrating the events of this transplant behind the scenes for years, and I had no clue. Once I traced the initial relationship back to its origin, I learned that God had been putting people in place across states (and continents) while establishing relationships dating back to the late 1940s for me to one day have a kidney transplant in 2018. God left no doubt in my mind that only He could orchestrate what happens past, present, and future. God's provision was the only reason I could have that kidney transplant—it was a heavenly opportunity, not a coincidence.

At the time of the call, I didn't think I was even healthy enough to have a transplant. One of the concerns my doctors had was related to my prostate. My prostate-specific antigen (PSA) numbers were high, and I was worried that I might get diagnosed with prostate cancer. If that diagnosis had taken place, I would not have been a candidate to receive the direct donation. Nor could I have received the transplant. Based on these factors, I didn't believe the medical staff would allow me to have another transplant because of the high risk of rejection.

Despite all these challenges, God directed my successful second transplant. He was able to bring all these conditions together for my good, even though, at times, I lacked the confidence that He would do so. Romans 8:28 NKJV speaks directly to this point: "And we know that all things work together for good to those who love God, to those who are called according to His purpose." Due to my testimony, I lean on that Scripture so much!

What's more, I had a consistent prayer partner while waiting for my second transplant. I already had an established prayer life during that time: praying every morning when I woke up and doing my devotionals for at least thirty minutes every day. However, utilizing the gift of praying with a partner was a difference-maker in my faith life. My partner and I strived to pray together at least three times weekly.

It is one thing to pray, but another thing to pray and watch how God answers—and He does so effortlessly. When I received the call from my sister, stating that there was a family who wanted to donate a kidney to me, I was in disbelief. God was *showing out* at this point!

The following day, I received a call from my donor coordinator at Johns Hopkins to discuss the status, process, timing, and what needed to be done to receive the kidney. After a lengthy conversation, she said, "Mr. Works, are you a praying man?" I responded, "Yes." She said, "Would you mind if I prayed with you?" I replied, "No, I don't mind!" She prayed with me that day, and we agreed in faith that a kidney was on the way. I am confident that she knew the kidney was compatible (or a match), and that there was a good chance that I would get the kidney, but she could share only so much at the time.

The fact that my donor coordinator reached out to me in prayer was God-ordained. By the time she finished praying, I was overcome with emotions. She didn't know me well, but she understood my story and was empathetic to my needs. My donor coordinator impacted me through her obedience to prayer and was another factor in my increased faith.

The timeline was this: I learned about a potential donor on Sunday; I prayed with my donor coordinator on Monday morning; Monday night, I was told the kidney was compatible; Tuesday night, I received a call from a nurse to come to the John Hopkins Hospital immediately; on Wednesday, I had the transplant. Considering how quickly and efficiently I received my second transplant, all I can say is, BUT GOD!

As I consider all the ways God has blessed me over my lifetime, I feel filled with humility. God has blessed me with not one but *two* kidneys. He blessed my wife with *two* successful pregnancies and *two* healthy daughters. When one job opportunity closed, He blessed me with not one new job offer but *multiple* offers. What is more, during that time, I met my annual sales objective in *four* months. God has been showering me with favor for a long time, and I am beyond thankful for His provisions. I had my last kidney transplant in 2018, and five years later, I still benefit from my God-given gift.

Lifestyle Changes

Recognizing that I've recovered from two transplants proves that no one is guaranteed a longstanding healthy life. Therefore, I've always known that a successful transformation would include maintaining the health of my kidneys—it was non-negotiable. I had to manage my eating habits, medications, and physical exercises to the best of my ability.

To illustrate, after my surgeries, my doctors told me that I could eat whatever I wanted in moderation. Though this may have been true, I was determined to consume only foods that would extend my life. Since then, I have been laser-focused on establishing good eating habits. I've also encouraged my loved ones to hold me accountable for my dietary goals.

To move forward physically, I needed to reevaluate what I consumed, the exercises I performed, and the overall treatment of my body. I had already committed to refrain from engaging in activities that would not prolong my life, such as smoking or drinking. This was because I was unwavering in my commitment to building a legacy for my wife and children.

In addition, I had to be willing to make some short and long-term life adjustments to maintain and extend the life of my new kidneys. Following my kidney transplants, my medical team recommended that I stay local within the first six months of my kidney transplant. The team also suggested that I refrain from leaving the country for work or vacation for at least one year.

In particular, my doctors recommended that I steer clear from vacationing on cruises. The challenge with cruises is that people are confined to a space where germs are overwhelmingly present—especially regarding buffet dining. Though there are perks of buffets, including self-service and variety, food can spoil quicker because it is kept at room temperature for an extended time. The longer food exceeds the proper temperature, the greater chance it can be exposed to germs that cause sickness. As a result, it was better that I avoid this source of entertainment altogether.

Coupled with certain activities, there are several types of foods that donor recipients are encouraged to avoid. Specifically, I was not supposed to eat undercooked foods like poultry, fish, raw seafood, unpasteurized cheeses, and eggs. So, I leaned towards getting my meats cooked well done, so there was a lesser chance of contamination. I didn't mind making these lifestyle changes because I knew they were minor in the big picture of life. If followed, these guidelines could enhance my chances of protecting my kidneys.

The most important consideration I want future organ recipients to know about lifestyle changes is that they must take preventative measures to prolong the life of the gift they have received. Adhering to these measures may mean missing out on exciting new opportunities along the way, but the reward is greater than the risks.

Philanthropic Growth

As an extremely blessed two-time kidney recipient, I have developed a very giving mindset. To think that people thought enough of me to get tested to become my organ donor has had a lasting effect on me. I may not be able to donate an organ, but I can and have identified charities and organizations that I will donate to for the balance of my years on this earth. Some organizations I have donated to are the United Negro College Fund, United Way, and the National Kidney Foundation, to name a few. I also contribute to my alma maters and educational foundations frequently because the funding that I provide to these institutions helps students afford higher education and better career opportunities.

In addition, I serve on the board of trustees of a very prestigious university and a few foundations. The goal behind my donations is to encourage and promote higher education for under-resourced students with the belief that I can create opportunities and aid in developing young minds. My goal is to use my skills to help each organization grow and contribute to its missions because I desire to make a long-standing impact on the less fortunate. God has blessed me tremendously across my career and the income-generating businesses that I have been able to establish. Therefore, I always seek opportunities to give back and bless others.

Empathetic Heart

I have experienced a transformation of my heart firsthand based on the trials I have overcome. Now, I have a very compassionate connection with those who may be going through similar healthcare challenges. When I attend appointments (sometimes lasting hours on end), I recognize that I am very fortunate to be alive.

As I previously mentioned, a person may wait four to five years to secure a kidney off the transplant list. The fact that I could secure kidneys for each of my transplants within eighteen months of my searches tells me that I am quite blessed. It is possible to secure a kidney from a live donor within a year if you have an extensive network and are aggressively reaching out to people to get tested—but it is no small feat. Getting a kidney off the transplant list can be a challenge on all fronts.

I have talked to people who have waited years to secure an organ off the transplant list. I am empathetic to their plight, especially because some people die while waiting for an organ transplant due to a shortage of available organs. Therefore, I do not take my blessings for granted and can relate to their pain. As I meet other donor recipients, I hear their stories, learn from their challenges, and understand and compare notes on what they are going through. I can relate to them because I have been there or know someone else who has had a similar experience. For example, shortly after I had been discharged from the hospital after my first kidney transplant, I learned of the passing of several individuals I had ties to directly or indirectly. Of those people, one was a patient whose manner of death impacted me greatly: he was a friend who had gone to the hospital for surgery and ended up having a blood clot. He died shortly after.

As I reflect on my friend's experience, the purpose of wearing those compression socks after surgery became very real. I wore a lightweight wrap around my legs in the hospital with intermittent compression. I was encouraged to wear them to increase circulation and protect against blood clots. Lying in bed and being sedentary for long periods of time can cause blood clots. This is a major reason why doctors want their patients up and walking after surgery. Thankfully, God protected me from having blood clots, but I sympathized with my friend's unfortunate passing because that could have been my reality.

Another death that impacted me shortly after my discharge was my childhood friend's daughter. At that time, this young lady was either going to or returning from an OBGYN appointment—she was expecting her first child. While driving, the tires on the back of a truck in front of her fell off and began bouncing on the highway. As a result, one of the tires smashed through her windshield and killed her on impact.

Tragedies such as these have influenced my testimony and made me appreciative for my organ-receiving experience. As these examples have shown, life is precious. We should not take for granted the borrowed time we have here on earth, and we should be empathetic toward the less fortunate.

Managing Grief

Over the years, I've learned that true transformation occurs in stages throughout various areas of life. When my mother passed away in January 2013, I experienced a profound season of grief. The time of her passing was between my first and second transplants, so coping with her death was naturally difficult because it caught my family by surprise.

I recall speaking at her funeral (which included nearly 1,000 attendees), overcome with emotions due to the outpouring of love from those around me. I looked at the faces in the church: her friends and family attended from across the country. Their faces were examples of the many lives she had touched when she was alive. It was then that I recognized that the illness that took her life would impact my family and me for the rest of our lives. It seemed unreal that we would never see her again.

The impact of her passing did not truly hit me until my daughter's third birthday party a week later. Her party was held at a gymnastics center. Every time the entry door opened, I couldn't help but longingly look for her. I was waiting for my mother to walk through the door, ready to celebrate her granddaughter's birthday. That is when it hit me that she was never coming back. This realization was probably one of the most challenging days of my life. It was a happy day to celebrate my daughter's birthday, but it was also distressing to recognize that my mother would no longer be physically present in our lives.

My mother's death was sudden and very traumatic, mainly because I was also struggling with kidney failure at that time. In response, I decided to undergo grief counseling with one of the pastors at my church for treatment. It was good for me to meet with him as I talked through the pain of losing my mother—taken from me like a thief in the night. Speaking with him helped me organize my thoughts from my emotions and get a better grasp on what I was going through. Overall, the counseling helped me a great deal.

During this time, I also stayed close to my father and was a strong support system for him. One of his closest friends reminded me I needed to give him space to adjust to the new normal without his wife. I received that advice. I knew that the chance of my father getting remarried was slim (he was seventy-nine years old at the time), so I wanted him to see that I was a confidant if he needed one. I also knew that no woman could take my mother's heart from him and no woman could have replaced her. He was content being by himself, and I was content accepting his grief for what it was. We built a stronger father-son relationship based on this mutual understanding.

When I meet people who have experienced the sudden death of a loved one, I can sincerely empathize with them. It is not easy to recover from the passing of someone you love and care about; it takes time, therapy, and patience to transform from a season of grief to a season of acceptance.

Dialysis Reality

I was first introduced to the possibility of dialysis as a treatment (sometime before my second kidney transplant) after I experienced an unexpected visit to the emergency room. During this follow-up appointment, I met with a doctor whose sole purpose was to eventually get me placed on dialysis. The doctor I was referred to shared the medical team's concern that my kidney functionality was declining rapidly. The physician told me they would no longer focus on my creatinine level; instead, they wanted to prepare me for dialysis within the next few months.

During the appointment, the doctor shared dialysis treatment options, the treatments details, and the dialysis preparation timeline. After his explanation, I began to warm up to the idea of dialysis. However, it didn't matter how I felt about the process. My options were limited: I would go on dialysis or suffer dire consequences. Considering I was relatively healthy (outside of end-stage renal failure) and in good shape, the doctors recommended the best form of dialysis for me would be peritoneal. This form of treatment could be administered at home, at night, and it was easier on my body.

Alternatively, having dialysis performed in-center would have been time-consuming. This method would take me away from my job anywhere from twenty-five to forty percent of each work week. If I had to go into a dialysis center to receive my treatments (three days a week, four hours at a time), there would be no way to guarantee how I would feel following the sessions. In addition, the travel time to and from the dialysis center for treatments would have been extensive. Being absent from my job forty percent of each week would have posed significant risks to my performance. In other words, it would have been harder to meet my goals if I had not been present.

After considering all my options, I decided to have a conversation with my boss. I told him that I could not perform my job and be on dialysis at the same time, no matter what dialysis option I selected. Therefore, I was going on long-term disability. At that time, I did not have a backup career plan, but I trusted that God would make a way to address my needs if ties to my current job were severed. Not long after this, God began to reveal other ways for me to address my financial needs that would support and meet most of my expectations.

In summary, I have experienced transformation in various forms: spiritual, mental, physical, and emotional. My transplants changed not only who I am internally but externally—they changed how I view the world. I've become a better person because of my trials and tribulations. These trials have stretched me as a person and have encouraged me to lean on God amid my battles. Consequently, I have increased patience while waiting for answers and guidance for life's next steps. As my end goals are met, I greatly appreciate having two successful transplants and two complete recoveries.

Chapter 10

NAVIGATING A PANDEMIC

After many years of transformation, in 2019, I was taken aback by the nation's response to the Coronavirus pandemic. If you are like me, initially, you were probably mildly annoyed and in disbelief regarding the severity of the virus. Eight weeks later, nearly forty million Americans filed for unemployment, and businesses were closing left and right. America's urban minority and rural communities began to take the hardest hits, and all the disparities came to the surface. The pandemic became a genie we could not put back into the bottle. There was much uncertainty as our lives were halted. Over the next few months, the United States lost over 100,000 people to COVID-related deaths.

Though information regarding the virus was making headlines, I wasn't influenced until late January 2020, when I talked to a friend at church. I had not seen this friend in over a year because his job required him to travel worldwide. His most recent overseas assignment was in China. He shared that he had just moved his family back to the United States due to the spread of COVID-19 in China. I did not know the seriousness of the virus at that time, but he had a firsthand taste. His employer recognized that the deadly virus was spreading, so the company sent him and his family back stateside. I understood then that some things do not become real until they impact someone you know.

COVID: Up Close and Personal

The week after this encounter, I had my bi-annual kidney appointment with my nephrologist. The feedback I received and the overall results from the visit were positive. My doctor was pleased with my progress. Almost two years had passed since my second transplant, and everything was going well. We did not discuss the COVID-19 virus or its symptoms during this visit. There were only a few cases in the United States at the time, and as it seemed, most people were not alarmed. However, the virus was becoming popular with infectious disease medical practitioners.

Over the next two months, the world as I once knew it would be forever altered. In March 2020, the World Health Organization (WHO) declared COVID-19 a pandemic. As a result, businesses began closing, schools moved from in-person to virtual, flights were canceled, and religious services were no longer held in person. The world had officially changed right before my eyes.

By the spring of 2020, medical facilities, hospitals, doctors, and nurses began to change how they administered patient services. The change was necessary to protect all medical providers, patients, and parties involved. Regarding immunocompromised patients, their protection and care went to an even higher standard. My medical team urged me to be vigilant, remain masked, monitor where I went, and refrain from frequenting crowded places. In addition, they shared that I should wash my hands thoroughly, sanitize all surfaces, and do everything to stay out of harm's way.

Organ recipient appointments were moved from in-person to virtual to reduce patients' exposure to people, germs, COVID-19, and other illnesses that could attack their immune systems. My doctors asked me to take my vitals at home and provide the results. My follow-up doctor's appointments were held virtually as well. Moving forward, Johns Hopkins Hospital leveraged video-conferencing technology to administer my appointments unless I had to visit the doctor in person. A few instances where an in-person meeting was required were for surgery or rehabbing an injury (like when I had surgery due to a physical injury).

In late November 2020, I had a series of doctor's appointments that would impact me for the next month. Before Thanksgiving, I visited the doctor to have my bi-monthly labs drawn; those lab results were in good standing. The following week, I had an MRI performed at another medical facility. The day before Thanksgiving, I called my transplant coordinator to discuss a few of my concerns about the MRI.

As a transplant patient, I first questioned whether it was even safe for me to have the MRI performed. For some reason, I thought that I should not be getting MRIs as a kidney transplant patient. The doctor stated, "No, you can have an MRI administered." Second, I had questions about a taste I had acquired since the imaging. When an individual undergoes an MRI, it is not uncommon to experience a metallic taste in their mouth. I later learned from my coordinator that this was not out of the ordinary. Third, I had a few side effects that I believed were related to the MRI; interestingly, they also mirrored symptoms of COVID.

When I brought these concerns to my transplant coordinator, he said, "Let me reach out to your nephrologist." After communicating with the coordinator, my nephrologist reached out to me and said, "You know, we've had several transplant patients that tested positive for COVID recently. Why don't you go ahead and get tested? Just to be safe." Based on his suggestion, my transplant coordinator scheduled my COVID test for the day after Thanksgiving. That day, I drove to the hospital and underwent my test. The next day, I was at home riding my stationary bike when I received a text. The text was from Johns Hopkins Hospital, where I had been tested; it stated that my results were POSITIVE.

Next Steps

Despite all the precautions I took to protect myself, I contracted COVID in November 2020. This was just a few months before the vaccine was rolled out to the general public. Testing positive was frustrating because I had been cautious everywhere I traveled within the Washington, DC, metro area. I wore gloves and masks in public and was double-masked most of the time. I ordered groceries online, had food delivered to my home, and disinfected food items before putting them away. In addition, I shopped during off-peak hours whenever I had the time to pick things up. Considering all the preventative care I took, I thought, "How did I catch COVID?"

My local health department called the day that I learned I tested positive. The representative began asking questions about my exposure and contact tracing. Attempting to comply, I traced my steps back a week, contacted the people I may have exposed, and let them know my test results and status. Everyone I spoke with got tested, and their results returned negative. That was a relief!

Next, I started asking questions related to a contractor that I had dealt with earlier that week. I was concerned that his mask may have slipped down when he was talking and that maybe he had accidentally exposed me to the virus. I wasn't entirely sure of this, though. After speaking to the contractor, I learned that he did not have COVID symptoms and was, therefore, not a virus carrier. At this point, I had no solid leads for my contact tracing.

Dealing with the conditions that resulted from the pandemic and testing positive became a major inconvenience. The results also burdened my wife significantly since she had to take full responsibility for the household duties: cooking, cleaning, doing laundry, and caring for our daughters.

In addition to this added weight, my daughters refrained from attending school during our quarantine and had to participate virtually via Zoom for two weeks. It was a challenging time, but looking back, I'm grateful for God's provision and the survival of our sanity.

Questions Answered and Major Changes

A week after I was notified of my positive test, I received a letter from the medical facility where my blood work and labs were taken. The letter shared that when I had been in to get my labs drawn, another party present was exposed to COVID-19. They did not say whether the person was a patient or an employee who had come into the facility and exposed me (this was to maintain that person's privacy). Nevertheless, the exposure required the facility to close for a few days for a thorough cleaning.

I can still play back the people present in the facility that day, as well as the medical practitioners who drew my blood and took my vitals. On that day, my world would change in minutes. As a result of the exposure, the medical facility immediately began doing its part to protect patients and employers.

As a reminder, pre-COVID, patients could make appointments online and participate in walk-in appointments freely; people sat in the lobby and were checked in and out by the assistants and practitioners. Today, most appointments are made online or via telephone. Medical facilitators respond via email with a confirmation of the appointment, confirmation number, and date and time. Next, patients click on the link sent to them to view confirmation, and the facility sends the patient a text requesting their notification upon arrival for said appointment. From there, the patient responds to the text letting the provider know they have arrived. Last, the medical facility responds with a text message informing patients that the medical practitioner is ready to see them.

From this point, the patient sits in the car (instead of the lobby) until the medical practitioner is prepared for the visit. This process allows the assistants to check in on the patient without human intervention and reduces contact. The assistant can provide the patient with a container for a urine sample during this process. The patient then goes to the bathroom, uses the container to catch urine, deposits the urine sample in the designated bathroom area, and goes directly to the physician's room to have additional lab work drawn. These streamlined activities have proven to reduce contact with personnel, shorten the time it takes to check a patient in and out, and accelerate the process of drawing labs.

One measure my medical team put in place was that they reduced the frequency I needed to have labs drawn. I used to get labs drawn monthly, but in the COVID era, my team reduced the number of times my labs were drawn to bi-monthly. The frequency of labs is drawn generally based on the patient's health. Fortunately, I was doing very well healthwise, and getting labs done bi-monthly was a non-issue.

Most modern-day patients are in and out of a medical facility within minutes—ten or less. My experience proved that it doesn't matter how long one is exposed or where they are; anyone can contract COVID at any time or place. I believe I did everything I could to protect myself from catching this virus, but I still tested positive. The exposure heightened my awareness of how I would approach the pandemic moving forward. I know that now more than ever, proper hygiene is essential.

Managing My Symptoms

Thankfully, the COVID symptoms I experienced were minor. However, I did experience a mild bout of diarrhea and an elevated temperature for twenty-four hours. Since I was already monitoring my vitals daily, when I began to feel ill, I knew there was a chance something was wrong. Still, I never thought for one minute that my symptoms were related to COVID. When my results came back positive, my transplant coordinator told me to quarantine for three weeks (due to my compromised immune system) versus the average ten days for people with no underlying health conditions.

While my experience with COVID was manageable, a very good friend who is also a kidney transplant patient was not as fortunate. After he tested positive, he told me that his COVID symptoms took a toll on him for days. He experienced a fever, chills, body aches, fatigue, and so much more. I knew that he had undergone quite a bit of suffering and that I should not complain about my more fortunate experience.

Even with the vaccine and booster shots, I know of organ recipients who have still tested positive for COVID and felt the weight of its symptoms. Regardless, kidney transplant patients or people with compromised immune systems must keep their guard up as it relates to COVID. While it may be difficult to see an end, remaining vigilant and prayerful during this time is the best course of action—this too shall pass.

Heightened Level of Cleanliness

The pandemic created phobias about germs and potential virus exposure in my household. As you know, I am immunosuppressed, but I also have a daughter with asthma. With little knowledge of the virus initially, my wife and I were focused on protecting our family. We were not taking any chances and were very cautious about what and who entered our home (in fact, we still are). Many people thought we were overreacting, but our family is still standing today despite their beliefs. That fact alone gives my loved ones and me great reassurance.

We took many steps to protect our home. These included, disinfecting surfaces, socially distancing, washing our hands, and wearing proper protective gear to reduce exposure to sickness. First, we established a *landing station* in a central location at the front entrance of our house. On the landing zone table, we placed proper protective gear such as hand sanitizer, masks, wipes, footies, and socks. Anytime my family entered our home, we immediately used them to sanitize.

Second, we did not let anyone (outside of our immediate family) enter our house during the first six to nine months of the pandemic. This practice ensured that the only people in our house were residents. Third, nine months after the pandemic started, we welcomed our first visitors. These visitors were essential contractors and cleaning service providers that enhanced the overall being of our nest.

Lastly, my wife and I cautiously allowed nonessential visitors to enter our home after becoming fully vaccinated in the summer of 2021. I use the term "vaccinated" cautiously because our youngest daughter was still not vaccinated at the time (the vaccine for children under 12 was not made available until the end of 2021).

In terms of handwashing, me and my family washed our hands just as I did when I was on dialysis, preparing for an exchange. Those steps included washing for a minimum of twenty seconds, scrubbing my hands thoroughly, and making sure to address all crevices. Every time we washed our hands, we also used hand sanitizer; this ensured that our hands were thoroughly disinfected and as clean as possible. Other steps we took included placing hand sanitizer in every bathroom and next to the kitchen sink at our home. We also encouraged our family members and guests to use these cleaning sources as often as possible. In addition, we kept hand sanitizer and disinfectant wipes in our cars to use as we came and went.

Additionally, I cannot express enough the importance of wearing a mask outside the home. Whenever I go out, I generally double-mask just as a safety precaution. Initially, I wore gloves when I shopped, but I have since reduced that practice. While shopping or going to the grocery store, I try to go at off-peak times because the stores are generally less populated. As you may know, stores and malls were shut down for some time. As a result, our family purchased items online. These were generally necessities that kept impulse purchases to a minimum.

More Proper Precautions

Outside of my heightened sense of cleanliness, I've also adjusted what activities I participate in since the emergence of COVID. To demonstrate, I have not returned to the gym since the pandemic began. The last day I entered a workout facility was the morning of March 11th, 2020. I remember asking my partner, "Is it me, or does the gym appear a little light today?" He responded, "It's light. It's been like this all week. It's due to COVID." As I watched ESPN on the monitor at the gym, the anchor announced that the NBA and NCAA college basketball tournament was canceled. I knew then that COVID was a big deal—the NBA & NCAA would not forgo losing millions of dollars if this pandemic was not real.

Ultimately, I decided to avoid working out at the gym because it is one of the riskiest places for catching COVID-19. People are sweating, touching multiple surfaces, breathing hard after exercises (without masks on), and near one another in a closed space; these were all major concerns for me. To clarify, I am not assuming that a person attending a gym will automatically be infected with the virus in that environment. However, I am saying that I wanted to take this location out of my exposure equation. Instead, I continued to exercise and work out at home. I began running outside, riding my bike, and lifting free weights to stay in shape as it got warm. Overall, I had to adjust how I approached exercise because of the pandemic.

Most importantly, I've always requested input from my medical team if I've had questions about anything that may impact my kidneys. Whenever I am asked to attend events, meetings, dinners, outings, and other activities, I run the requests by my medical team. I want to secure their guidance on whether it is safe to attend the event and, if not, understand their rationale. I've noticed that their recommendations two months before an event can change over time because of COVID's fluidity. Nonetheless, I depend on my medical staff to share the most updated information on proper precautions.

For example, activities in old buildings with poor ventilation have been a non-starter for me. Though buildings in this condition may be getting cleaned, if they lack proper air circulation, there is a major cause for concern. Indoor events with a large flow of people in attendance are also off-limits. In addition, when I am invited to events, I always question whether hand sanitizer, gloves, and masks will be made available for use. Sometimes these factors are not present, so I abstain from participating rather than attending these events and risk my health. Events with large crowds in uncontrolled environments have far too much risk for me to be in attendance.

It's more vital for me to forgo temporary pleasure than to make a mistake that could cause long-term health issues. As a result, I have since declined attendance at major sporting or entertainment events while the virus rages. While the requirement may be for attendees to adhere to a mask mandate, people have gotten lax as time has gone by, and I can't afford to risk their lack of caution. Some people are tired of wearing masks and believe they are untouchable until someone they know gets exposed to the virus, gets really sick, or passes away.

However, I have allowed my family and me to partake in the viewing of smaller sporting events. My children attend a K-12 school, and I've taken them to some football games because they are less populated. When I attend athletic events, I stand away from the crowd. This way, I am in more control of my environment and away from crowded spaces. I won't have to worry about someone speaking to me (especially if they haven't been practicing social distancing) or coming in contact with someone (because they're in my space) if I have additional space between us. This approach has allowed me to move forward in the COVID environment.

Difficult Conversations

Amid the pandemic, I have had difficult conversations with some family members and loved ones regarding my event attendance. These events may include family dinners, school events, church, funerals, games, plays, and many other activities. Most people are understanding, but others have been offended when I have declined their requests. In response, I was not concerned about what they thought. I knew my preventative actions were protecting my family. I could not stress whether someone's feelings would be hurt based on how I responded to their invitation.

My situation was different: my actions could keep me at home with my family or place me on a respirator. Therefore, I chose the former. I watched relatives, and close family friends get exposed to the virus, battle the virus, and subsequently pass away. Some had pre-existing conditions, while others did not. Still, it was clear that the virus attacked people with weak immune systems particularly harshly. My goal was to protect and be there for my family for as long as possible.

Granted, the situations I am referring to all happened prior to the approval of the COVID-19 vaccine. After a recent conversation with my transplant coordinator, I learned that hospitals were still experiencing a rise in COVID cases—even from people who had been vaccinated and boosted. Whenever I hear about someone being affected by the pandemic, becoming really sick, or passing away, my conversations with others are more straightforward.

Ultimately, COVID has touched people from all walks of life and businesses. Specifically, in 2020, funeral organizers pivoted from their traditional approach to better address the needs of their clients. Funeral homes began to offer valuable services, including streaming and outdoor ceremonies. These options were made available because of government-mandated COVID restrictions, such as strict capacity limits. Before this, a lack of social distancing at funerals was a breeding ground for the COVID-19 viral spread.

I know more than a handful of people who have gone to funerals and been exposed to the virus. For example, my friend attended a funeral last year during the holiday season. He told me that after participating, nearly a dozen funeral attendees tested positive for COVID. His feedback reiterated what I already knew to be true: I did not need to attend *any* crowded events.

Another example of funeral exposure was when my close friend attended a funeral out of town. Family and friends flew in for the funeral from different parts of the country. Although it was a small service and attendance was low, one of the family members was exposed to the virus by an out-of-town guest. Subsequently, she tested positive, went from experiencing mild symptoms to severe illness, and passed away. Due to fatal incidents such as this, I'm not swayed to attend certain activities because I recognize the life-threatening exposures of this virus. I approach these scenarios at my own risk, so I always consult with my doctors about the potential complications beforehand.

During a pandemic, family gatherings around the holidays can also be a complex subject to discuss. My family is no different. Sometimes, in preparation of these functions, not all planning details are divulged. This past year, Thanksgiving dinner was held at two separate houses: my home and my sister's. First, my father, one of my sisters, and my nephew came to my house. Then, my father, sister, and nephew went to my sister's house. Though this was not an ideal situation, we were very conscious of the spread of the virus at the time and felt that this was the best course of action.

Our Christmas dining experience was a little different. Initially, we planned to hold Christmas dinner together, with both families eating at my father's house. My dad wanted to host the meal so that we could cook at his home. My sister, who resides in the same area as me, shared that her family was going out of town on vacation the week before Christmas and returning on Christmas Eve. My family and I were uncomfortable with her travel arrangements, especially so close to our upcoming family meal. So, after much thought, we came to a compromise. I recommended that my family eat dinner with my father on Christmas and my sister's family eat dinner with him on New Year's. Although it was a great compromise, it did not transpire as planned.

Later that December, one of my relatives fell under the weather. As a precaution, they decided to take a COVID test. When their results came back positive, my family decided to adjust our New Year's Day dinner plans accordingly. We could not risk gathering and potentially exposing each other to illness. Of course, we were disappointed to cancel the event, but our health was the utmost priority. This situation is yet another example of why it is important to place your health in front of fellowship and fun.

When I look at the concept of family gatherings during a pandemic, I understand that it only takes one carrier to infect a whole party. When I hear people say, "Oh, well, we're vaccinated, and we also received the booster shot," I am still not moved. These people fail to realize that they can still contract COVID regardless of their vaccination status. Irrespective of their vaccination status, people that fail to exercise proper precautions are more likely to increase the spread of germs. Furthermore, I believe that I cannot depend on others to advocate for my health. I must focus on what's suitable for me because if something tragic happens, my absence will harm my family. I don't want my loved ones to experience the pain and mourning of losing me. Therefore, I try to protect myself from illness to reduce the chance of a health-related death.

Church

One of the leading institutions affected by the COVID-19 pandemic was the church. I am a member of a congregation with over 10,000 members attending services each Sunday. Our sanctuary holds approximately 4,500 people. Before the pandemic, we held four services each Sunday: 8:00 a.m., 10:00 a.m., noon, and 6:30 p.m. We have over one hundred plus ministries and we naturally met in person. However, during the pandemic, our congregation was able to pivot immediately.

The Sunday before we closed the doors of the church, we were doing fist bumps versus shaking hands and hugging to greet our fellow parishioners. Hand sanitizer stations were placed around the church as safety measures. The following week, our service was streamed online and held virtually. The operation was established and delivered so professionally that it appeared a major network on television was producing our service.

I commend my pastor because he placed safety first to ensure our parishioners were not impacted negatively by COVID. He held steadfastly and studied the scientific results; he listened to the health experts and the local county and state officials before making plans or announcements about returning to the sanctuary. He developed a two-step process to re-enter our sanctuary in the fall of 2021: a tent revival and services held outdoors for three Sundays before returning indoors. However, due to an uptick in the number of COVID cases in our region, we couldn't fully transition back into the church. So, he pivoted once again.

I appreciate a man of God being Spirit-led on when to open the church and resume services. Living with a compromised immune system, I know my pastor was concerned about members with health challenges, such as myself. He did not want to lose any members or guests because he reopened our church doors too early.

My church returned to in-person services in April 2022. The Sunday schedule was changed to offer services at 9:00 a.m. and 11:30 a.m. each Sunday, and on fourth Sundays, we have our Communion Service at 6:30 p.m. Between services, cleaning specialists disinfected the sanctuary. In addition to this, to limit sickness exposure, we continued to offer Sunday services online. Sunday school meets in a hybrid format through in-person and virtual learning. All ministry leaders and those participating in the service must be tested for COVID the week before serving. The goal is to make the environment as safe as possible as parishioners return to the sanctuary. In my eyes, this represents the model for how to re-enter a church after a pandemic effectively. This process helped me immeasurably in my decision to participate in in-person services.

Career

Navigating a pandemic sometimes requires adjusting to the transition. When COVID shut down access to most nonessential business activities, my job was one of the first to transition virtually. For some time after that, I worked from home. Now, you may be wondering, "Have you been back in the office since the rise of the pandemic?" The answer to that question is "Yes." I have returned to the office to pick up supplies and receive technical support. However, these are generally short visits; they may last five to ten minutes, and I may see only a couple of people tops. If I have to get my computer fixed, naturally, I interface with the computer technician.

I believe that my employer did a commendable job of helping employees navigate the pandemic. My employer put requirements in place before employees could enter the building. First, we had to upload our vaccination cards to the company system in advance and use our key-card to enter our office. Once staff members enter the office, use of the hand sanitizer stations are encouraged, and masks are mandatory to wear. Plexi-glass has been put in place in multiple areas to create additional protection from germs among staff. These preventative measures aim to protect personnel.

The initial precautions my employer took provided comfort to our workplace. Though there are very few people in the office today, for now, things appear safer than they were before the pandemic. Overall, our offices are much less populated because many jobs have been reclassified from in-office to virtual. However, once the office becomes more populated, we will better understand the comfort level our colleagues have working in the office.

Additionally, I have not physically been in front of a customer in over two years. That is because most of my customers operate in a hybrid mode if they return to their offices. Some of my customers have shared that their team members reside in different cities across the country, so leveraging technology is the most efficient means to meet. My customers pivoted to Microsoft Teams, Zoom applications, and other forms of video communication through modern technology. The adoption of these platforms has increased tenfold since the arrival of COVID. Individuals can hold virtual meetings, collaborate via instant messaging, place phone calls from a computer, schedule meetings online, and collaborate conveniently with co-workers from the comfort of their homes.

Similarly, some of my co-workers have returned to the office in a hybrid format while many are considering their options. I have not heard of many employee positions returning to the office five days a week. Ultimately, it doesn't seem as if the absence from the office has hindered our ability to work with customers. Though the virus has changed how people do business, most would say the changes are advantageous. In today's age, consumers have learned how to share information effectively, anytime and anywhere—everyone has the potential to navigate and conduct business amid a global pandemic.

The technology that arose before and during the pandemic also aided in my job security. My business was able to stay operational partly because employees were able to maintain their roles outside of the office. The work-from-home feature was especially beneficial for me as a two-time kidney recipient. Working from home reduced my exposure to the virus, all while I stayed productive in the virtual workplace. I couldn't have asked for a better setup than that.

Dining

At the beginning of the pandemic, the "dining in" experience was eliminated from all restaurants. Carry-out and pick-up options for food became the norm and kept many businesses afloat. Still, some did not make it based on these methods and had to close their doors permanently. My family's experience was consistent with the general population: we ordered carry-out. We picked up food as a substitute for the restaurant experience.

As the government relaxed its mandates and opened the economy up for business, restaurants were some of the first businesses to benefit from the *great reopening*. Restaurants began opening at twenty-five to fifty percent of their capacity. Some established outdoor seating in parking lots to expand their reach and create a new dining experience. I tended to favor dining outdoors because on rare occasions, that was the best option for me.

Since the pandemic, I have dined at a restaurant four times over the past two years. Two of those occasions were in the summer of 2021, and they were at restaurants where I could dine outside. Back then, my friends were sensitive to my concerns about eating inside and ensured we had a table away from the crowd. The people at my table wore masks but naturally removed them when we ate or drank. I was well aware of the consequences dining may have and the potential exposure from patrons removing their masks to eat. However, I felt comfortable dining in that environment.

Later that summer, I was on the committee of an organization hosting a gala. The event would be one where we estimated approximately 250 to 300 people would be in attendance. However, the numbers were scaled back significantly due to uneasiness regarding the pandemic. As a committee member, I questioned whether the event should be held, the attendance results, the financial statistics from ticket sales, and most importantly, how we would pull this off during the pandemic. By this time, businesses had reopened, but people were still practicing social distancing. Considering these factors, the hotel assured my team that they could accommodate a socially distanced event. Additionally, waiters would serve guests at their tables (versus buffet style), masks were mandatory, and proof of vaccination would be enforced.

Months in advance, I reached out to my medical team and asked if I could attend the gala. At the beginning of the summer, the number of Coronavirus cases had declined. In response, my providers responded that I could attend the event. They provided a caveat for me to reach out to them a couple of weeks before the event to see if things had changed with the pandemic.

A few weeks before the gala, I had my in-person bi-annual follow-up appointment. My lab work was good, and they provided me the nod to attend. After my appointment, I was asked to participate in a clinical trial to determine if I had antibodies to fight off the virus. Many doctors and patients were concerned because there was an ongoing study of transplant patients getting vaccinated and tested for antibodies. The results showed that most patients did not contain any antibodies, so they were not protected against the virus. After getting tested for antibodies, my results showed that I had antibodies at the level of a person without underlying health conditions: this was great news. My results indicated that I did not qualify for the trial because they were looking for patients that did not have antibodies.

However, as I talked to the nurse administering the trial, she was greatly concerned. I had shared my desire to attend this gala before being tested for antibodies, and her response was, "Let's get the results before I weigh in on whether you should attend or not." Once I received my results, she asked questions that I believed were second nature: "How many people will be attending the event? Is proof of vaccination required? Will masks be enforced? Will people be eating and drinking at the gala?" At this point, I was dumbfounded. Will people be eating and drinking at a gala? What kind of question was that!? I responded, "Yes…that is what people do at a formal dinner."

At that moment, the nurse shared her concerns about exposure to the virus because people would take off their masks to eat and drink. She said that ventilation and air circulation would be good in the ballroom and that an estimated 250 to 300 guests (in a room that typically holds over 1,000 people seated) should provide adequate social distance. Yet, the matter remained that the space was *indoors*.

At this stage in time, the country was changing. The new variant, Delta, was increasing at an alarming rate, and hospital visits were raging. Due to these circumstances, the nurse recommended that I forgo attending the gala. After consulting with my medical team, they concurred with her recommendation. So, I decided not to attend the event.

Looking back, I am grateful that I followed the advice of my medical advisors. This event occurred in the summertime when the pandemic started to chart record-high cases. If I had been in attendance, I might have been exposed to COVID. I later learned that safety protocols were relaxed after people arrived at the gala. In fact, I know of a few people that left because they felt uncomfortable in that environment. Fortunately, though, no one got sick, and the event was well received overall. I know a few people who shared that they would have walked me out of the event if I had attended. It's relieving to know that I have friends that care about my well-being, and I appreciate their concern more than they know.

Home Management

As mentioned, significant precautions must be taken to minimize exposure to potential virus carriers as organ recipients. In 2022, nationwide school districts and states are telling students and staff that the mask mandate is being lifted. My children are currently in middle school. Following this announcement, they brought their concerns to my attention. One of my daughters said, "Daddy, did you know that on March 8th, the school is lifting the mask mandate restriction? That means that we will have the option to attend school and not wear masks." She continued, "Daddy, you know what? I will still wear my masks because I believe more people will start testing positive for COVID." My other daughter then said, "Me too! I am trying to protect myself. I don't want to get COVID."

Even though both of my daughters are now vaccinated, they wanted to ensure they took advantage of all the proper precautions to avoid sickness. This dialog with my daughters confirmed that my conversations with them at home had not been in vain. I knew that dedication to preventing virus exposure had seeped into my family because even my daughters were on board with preventive planning.

Though my situation proved fruitful, I am aware that may not be the case for other organ recipients who have older children in their households. Teenagers may respond differently to COVID safety recommendations because they are often subjected to outside influences and peer pressure. Some may feel they are not at risk—as if they are invincible and that the pandemic rules don't apply to them. This may also present challenges for households with multiple teenagers who are used to coming and going as they please. As a parent, my recommendation for these young people is that they humble themselves and realize that this ongoing pandemic has serious consequences for people of all ages. Considering everything you've read so far, it is clear that COVID shows no favoritism: it is lethal to old and young people.

Travel

I have been very cautious about traveling during the pandemic. Per my doctor's recommendation, I have not traveled out of town since February 2020. It makes for a pretty dull life staying in one location for over two years, but overall, I have been safe from sickness.

When travel was necessary, I consulted with my doctors several times, asking for safety guidance; this was to attend board meetings, vacations, or engage in other work-related trips. For in-person conferences, the first question my doctors would ask is, "Is there an option for you to attend remotely?" If that option was available, my doctors generally preferred that form of attendance.

In addition to out-of-town travel, to date, I have not driven my car with anyone outside of my immediate family. I have made this decision because my preferred method of transportation is self-driving; I want to make sure I can control the environment I am operating in. As a result, I have not ridden a plane, train, or bus since the onset of the pandemic. When traveling, I allow my daughters to remove their masks when they get in my vehicle. They are offered hand sanitizer and disinfectant wipes to use as often as needed. They represent my environment and space, so naturally, we feel comfortable around one another.

When we stop for gas, I wear a mask and use gloves to pump. Afterward, I remove my gloves and properly disinfect my hands by hand washing or sanitizer. Then, I use a disinfectant wipe to wipe down all heavily touched areas, such as the steering wheel, doors, mirror, and cup holders. I'm almost germophobic now.

Pre-COVID, I never thought I would be taking the preventative measures I do now. However, as a two-time kidney transplant survivor, I know that these steps are necessary to decrease the spread of viruses. Wherever I go, I make sure to establish healthy boundaries so that I can ensure my safety. These procedures have become like second nature as I navigate the COVID-19 pandemic.

Chapter 11

LIFE FOREVER CHANGED

Many assume that the most challenging part of my journey was the kidney transplant surgery itself. Though the surgery was a critical component, it was not the most difficult, for anything temporary can be tolerated most times.

There is a checklist of things that happen before, during, and after the transplant process, and I will discuss them in this chapter. I was certainly better prepared for my kidney transplant the second time because I had already experienced it once before. However, one factor unsettled me for a long time—the reality that my life was forever changed.

Accepting Change

After my diagnosis, my life changed when I understood that my medications were not optional. While many people struggle with this fixed fact, most people recovering post-transplant learn to accept the large variety of prescribed medications. A few common ones are:

- Immunosuppressants (anti-rejection)
- Angiotensin-converting enzyme (ACE) inhibitors

- Anti-infectives
- Gastro-intestinal drugs (GIs)
- Vitamins/electrolytes
- Blood pressure medications

I mention these prescriptions because no matter what type of illness you are diagnosed with, the reality is that for some, taking medication is the difference between life and death. Even in cases where the lack of medication does not equate to fatality, the uncertainty of not taking designated prescriptions often dictates the quality of life. To the dismay of many, some medicines are only taken for a limited period. For example, I know people who tried to manage their diagnosis without taking the medication as prescribed. They ended up in a place where their circumstances changed, their health declined, the previous medications were no longer effective, and some eventually passed away.

As previously stated, following the doctor's orders is vital because taking matters into your hands can prove fatal. Although the reality of taking daily medications can be stressful, you must embrace your new lifestyle. Do not think for one minute that you do not have to take your medication—even when you are feeling good. Taking your medications generally has a direct impact on how you feel. Below are a few steps to better accommodate yourself to these medical changes:

1. *Find people who are fighting the same illness that you are.*

Sometimes the best people to help you go through a struggle victoriously are the same people who are already in the ring fighting their enemy. I found understanding through online support groups for kidney recipients on Facebook and Yammer. The posts on these sites allowed me to ask questions, share news, and gain encouragement throughout my journey. They helped me realize that I was not alone. I considered them to be my online community—family that I could lean on. If you are struggling with accepting the conditions of your diagnosis, there are all kinds of in-person or virtual groups available. You can also seek out local nonprofits and churches that may offer this type of support.

2. *Be okay with having "health-essential" boundaries.*
COVID-19 made all of us adjust to a "new normal." That "normal" is even more challenging for people with pre-existing health conditions. My family was highly at-risk for Coronavirus. While adjusting to the rest of the changes in the world, I made lifestyle transformations that were difficult for my co-workers and family to understand. However, I could not worry about offending anyone at that time. Instead, I created an elevator "pitch" to educate everyone on how I had to function during the pandemic to keep myself safe.

3. *Be ready to redesign your life…again…and again.*
Being flexible during your journey will aid in your strength. I sought out a nutritionist; she was essential in helping me maintain a healthy diet. Another activity that I embraced was exercise. Running and lifting light weights helped maintain my health. When I ran for the first time after being down for six months, I was figuratively a fish out of water. My legs grew very tired, and I felt relatively weak. Yet, over time, I persevered, bounced back, and was in fighting shape.

4. *Choose joy.*
Happiness is a choice. Having a life-changing medical diagnosis is not anything most people would choose. Still, you have to embrace the unique opportunity to live your life on your terms. I want to encourage you to do just that. Though accepting that you have a life-changing illness may be tough initially, if you follow the guidelines, you can still live a successful, fruitful life.

Adjusting to Dialysis

As mentioned in the earlier chapter, despite all the precautions I took to stay healthy, I eventually had to adjust to dialysis. My condition declined for the worse prior to my second transplant. It was a spring day on March 31, 2017. I remember the day specifically because it was my company's last day of the quarter (which had been very stressful for me). After leaving a client's office, I went to the hospital to get an Epogen shot: a shot that I had been taking regularly, a couple of times a month, to increase my red blood cell count.

The process involved a nurse taking my blood pressure. If my blood pressure fell within the acceptable range, the nurse would administer the shot. My blood pressure was extremely high that day—this was a first for me. I thought that maybe the change was because of the stress I was facing at work. My systolic number (the first blood pressure number) was over two hundred. The medical staff checked this measurement several times over the next ninety minutes, but the systolic number would not budge.

The nurse informed me that my blood pressure was at what medical professionals considered a "stroke level." When one experiences blood pressure readings greater than 180:120, they are at a high risk of having a stroke. To translate, I was having a hypertensive crisis. What's odd is that I wasn't feeling bad at all. However, once the nurses realized my blood pressure wasn't coming down, they shared that I could not leave the hospital and needed to be taken to the Emergency Room (ER). Upon entering the ER, I was immediately taken into a room for evaluation. After getting assessed, the nurse shared that I had two problems: first, my blood pressure was extremely high, and the medical staff could not reduce it. Second, my creatinine level was elevated and was continuing to rise.

The doctors and nurses had combed through all my medical records by this time. As I lay in the ER bed, the nurse stated, "You will not be leaving the hospital any time soon. At least not until things are under control. If we had a kidney donor for you today, we would perform the transplant immediately." Apparently, my physical condition was that severe.

The medical staff also informed me that they wanted to place me on dialysis while I was in the hospital. Hearing that news caused me to panic. Remember, my mother collapsed right after having dialysis treatment. She passed away shortly afterward as the doctors could not revive her. Accepting the same treatment was not interesting to me, nor did I appreciate being notified of the necessity on such short notice. Fortunately, I did not have to go on dialysis that day, but by the fall of 2017, I was indeed placed on dialysis. The method employed was peritoneal dialysis. By way of digression, there are different methods:

1. Hemodialysis: a form of therapy where the patient can go in-center to a kidney dialysis center. The dialysis treatment is performed here three times per week, four hours at a time, or it can be performed outpatient from your home for 5 to 6 days a week, 2.5 to 3 hours per treatment. This dialysis aims to purify the blood of a patient whose kidneys are not working normally. During this process, the blood is filtered outside of the body through a dialyzer to remove unwanted waste, toxins, and excess fluids.

2. Peritoneal: a procedure performed at a patient's home every day, generally at night, for eight to ten hours per treatment. Before implementing therapy, a catheter is surgically placed into one end of the abdomen, extending outward from the skin on the other and allowing the patient to perform the dialysis treatment. This process removes excess fluid, corrects electrolyte problems, and removes toxins in those with kidney failure. It can be conducted manually or by being connected to a machine. This treatment serves the same purpose of taking excess fluid from your body and is less intrusive.

3. <u>Hemofiltration</u>: generally performed at a dialysis center but can also be performed at home. The patient will typically go to the center three times per week, and the therapy runs three to five hours. This therapy is used to treat acute kidney injury. During this process, a patient's blood is passed through a set of tubing via a machine to a semipermeable membrane where waste products and water are removed by convection. Replacement fluid is added, and the blood is returned to the patient.

Depending on a patient's medical state, a doctor will generally decide which form of dialysis is best for them and their lifestyle.

Other factors that contributed to my dialysis experience. For instance, when I was enduring these treatments, I had no dietary restrictions. My nurse directed me to begin my dialysis treatments simultaneously every night. As such, I established a window of time when I would start because getting connected and disconnected from the machine was a process. It could take over ten hours to get connected, perform the exchanges, and get disconnected.

Overall, the process taught me that it is essential to be flexible before you have a transplant, during dialysis, and afterward. Though I was initially hesitant to receive dialysis, I knew that the process was necessary for me to move forward in my transplant journey.

Chapter 12

STAY THE COURSE (THE CHRONIC ILLNESS MARATHON)

As a two-time kidney recipient, I have received news that has been less than promising as it relates to my kidney situation. Whether it was delivered by a doctor, donor coordinator, transplant coordinator, or potential donor, learning how to navigate past negativity has become one of my strengths. In this chapter, I will similarly teach you how to stay the course while running the chronic illness marathon laid before you.

Potential Donors

As I was trying to identify potential donor candidates, I received mixed results and feedback from the people I targeted. Some donor candidates stepped forward without being asked to get tested; some did not respond, and some agreed to get tested after I sat down and talked with them about the process. After this initial agreement, some proceeded with the next step by contacting my medical team to immerse themselves in the process. Others sat back and waited for me to re-initiate my request before they acted.

I quickly learned that people use various communication methods to convey their messages. Some of the most disheartening feedback I received from potential donors was nonverbal—it's less about what they said and more about their actions (or lack thereof). After I made second and third calls to potential donor candidates, sometimes those calls were returned, and sometimes they weren't. A few people would give me the run-around, saying they would get tested when they had no plans. Others would say, "Hey, look, you know, I spoke to my wife, and I'm waiting for her to respond." Later, I would learn they had never reached out to their spouse to discuss getting tested.

These instances were common among some friends and family—people I believed I would have no problems counting on to be transparent and helpful. Although this deception was not the case for all my candidates, a couple delivered one excuse after another, delaying the decision-making process. At that point, I realized that if I had to chase a person down for them to consider being my donor, then they were not the right person for my cause.

Despite their uncertainty, I also understood that some people did not know how to say "No," some did not want to hurt my feelings, and others may have feared the operation. I recognized that, in many respects, their responses were naturally humane. Although people may agree to commitments at first, at the end of the day, some are just not dependable. Initially, I struggled with this life lesson but understood it much better as time passed.

For my second transplant, I took the same approach to secure donors. Unfortunately, when I went through this process, my first compatible candidates could not be donors this time around. One person's medical situation changed, while another donor candidate worked through their family's medical challenges. I understood this friend's dilemma and encouraged her to focus on her loved one versus myself. I would never put myself before a friend's family member. I believed and knew I would secure a kidney from *someone*; I just didn't know who that *someone* would be.

After donor searching for over a year, I couldn't believe I had several leads for potential donors but no viable candidates. Though I had people willing to get tested, there was not a single prospect that had been through the initial work-up and was successfully moving through the screening process. This lack of initiative was alarming to me, but being honest, I was still in the beginning stages of securing a donor. It wasn't long after that I would receive a call that would change my life for the better.

My sister called me one afternoon and said that someone she and her husband knew wanted to direct a kidney to me. The reality of this offer was overwhelming. Initially, I held the phone in my hand, too amazed to speak. In my desperate search to secure my second donor, God had once again shown up right…on…time. This phone call was not a coincidence; instead, it was confirmation that *God is real.*

As I've often said, "Securing a kidney donor is not a sprint; it's a marathon." My situation taught me that recipients should always look at numerous opportunities to accomplish their endgame; who knows who the potential donation source could be. In hindsight, I remember my mother telling me that she was never concerned about me finding a donor. She always believed that would not be a problem for me; she knew God was in control, and now, so do I.

Doctors and Medical Staff

I didn't experience many challenges with my doctors during my transplants. As they monitored me post-transplant, they shared new information as they cared for me. When I battled viruses and had biopsies to evaluate the health of my kidney, they effectively assessed my medical condition and made necessary recommendations.

To reiterate, six years after my first transplant, my doctors told me I would need a second kidney one day. Initially, I saw this as a significant setback; that is, until I learned the average useful life of a transplanted kidney. If a person had received a transplant from a live donor, the average useful life of the transplanted kidney would be 10 to 15 years, *if* there were no setbacks.

Unfortunately, I had battled a virus, experienced scarring of my kidney tissue, and my body did not respond favorably to a full dose of one of the anti-rejection medications. Though my doctor wanted me to keep my kidney for ten years, that wishful thinking proved to be a stretch. For a person that obtained their kidney from a cadaver or deceased person, the average useful life use would be up to 10 years. These were all factors I had to consider when accepting the source of my kidney donation.

In my eyes, the statistical data provided was not favorable or unfavorable—it was *real*. I wasn't aware of this information before my first transplant, and if I had been, I'm not sure how I would have responded to the knowledge. I believe my doctors didn't share this detail with me because they were trying to get me to the finish line without alarming me.

The reality of a kidney's useful life could be disturbing from a recipient's perspective, but from a front-row seat, I welcomed the transparency. I was unhappy about the delay in receiving this information over the years. I wanted to understand what I was dealing with to provide input into my treatment plan—I felt that this information would help me stay the course. Knowing the useful life of my kidney allowed me to discuss with my medical team the plan that eventually got me to my second transplant.

I was also told that I could live comfortably with my creatinine level at its current state for a few years. The downside of this is that I would eventually become anemic, and my red blood cell count would decline. Then, my condition would require bi-weekly hospital visits to secure

Epogen shots that would increase my hemoglobin levels. Without these shots, I would experience fatigue regularly.

Simultaneously, around this time, my medical team discussed whether dialysis would be necessary. My nephrologist wanted to avoid dialysis and only use that treatment as a last resort. However, after the incident I mentioned in the last chapter landed me in the hospital, a port was placed in my chest, and dialysis was administered immediately. At that time, my condition eventually stabilized, and my doctors didn't have to proceed with that procedure. However, over the next five months, my kidney functionality began to decline; this led to my transition to my long-term dialysis.

After I went on dialysis, there became a greater sense of urgency to secure a donor. I viewed this procedure as a means to an end—it served as a bridge to my transplant. It took me five months to secure a kidney, but my nurses cheered me on throughout the process. They were a source of encouragement I will never forget. As I share my testimony, I know God had His hand on me as I ran the chronic illness marathon.

Overcoming Hurdles

I've seen different things that give me hope related to longevity with kidney transplant patients. I have watched some people experience multiple transplants and overcome their health woes. In addition, social media offers a wealth of information about kidney disease survivors and their success stories. I know and have read about people who have had organ failure and waited on the transplant list for five-plus years. Others have been on dialysis for over twenty years and still live healthy lives.

I am encouraged by these stories because they reaffirm what I've believed in God for: favor and long life. My prayer is that my second kidney transplant will carry me for thirty-plus years. My experience has taught me that it doesn't matter how many transplants a patient may undergo; with the proper medical attention and resources, a recipient can make a full recovery.

I would encourage anyone in my situation to stay the course and never give up in their donor search. For example, a few days after Christmas in 2021, I received a call from my sister-in-law stating that someone she knew in Dallas, TX, had passed away, and their family was trying to donate the organs. They were trying to identify people that needed an organ so it could be directed to them as soon as possible. Fortunately, I identified two people, one of which was my sister, who was determined to take advantage of this Christmas gift. Each person provided me with their personal information in a matter of minutes. I forwarded that information to my sister-in-law's connection, and they submitted it to the doctors managing the process.

Two days later, both were notified that their blood type was either a match or compatible with the organs. That meant that the doctors would be moving forward with their transplants. Each person was told to go to the hospital the following day to be admitted. Both patients were shocked at how quickly things moved, were grateful to receive the gift of life, and were excited about their upcoming opportunities.

On the same day, both organs were sent from Dallas, TX, to hospitals in the Baltimore/Washington, DC, metropolitan area. As each patient was finalizing preparations for surgery, they began receiving results from their final tests. Shortly thereafter, I received a call from my sister stating that she tested positive for COVID. The following day, I received the same message from the other transplant candidate.

Though neither candidate was able to receive a kidney that day, fortunately, those kidneys did not go to waste. At each hospital, the next candidates on the kidney transplant list became the recipients of those organs. When I shared this incident with others, some asked why the doctors couldn't save the kidneys for the original two recipients when they recovered from COVID. This is because organs must be transplanted within a certain period before they are no longer viable.

Each of the previously mentioned transplant candidates was disappointed because the organ donation opportunity passed them. They were shocked they tested positive for COVID but later contact-traced their exposure to the virus. Furthermore, each candidate had successful kidney transplants over the next two months. Today, they are both doing well and back to living normal lives.

These examples demonstrate the importance of waiting on the Lord. I believe that when a person prays to God, He generally answers in one of three ways: yes, no, or not at this time. Additionally, it is beneficial for us to lean on Psalm 27:13,14 NKJV, "I would have lost heart, unless I had believed that I would see the goodness of the Lord in the land of the living. Wait on the Lord; be of good courage, and He shall strengthen your heart; wait, I say, on the Lord!"

In God's eyes, those kidneys were not for the people we thought they were designated for; instead, God had two others in mind. Furthermore, we serve a "right on time" God. He proved His timely deliverance when He addressed these individuals' needs a few months later.

These situations happened amid the COVID pandemic in December 2021 as exposure to the virus was raging. By the latter part of February, each original candidate had experienced successful kidney transplants. God made it possible for each of them to have their transplants, and I believe He can do the same for you. Though they couldn't use the kidneys offered in one season, the Lord blessed them with organs in another. Their stories are confirmation that although we cannot always control the timing of our needs, God will deliver results in the season He believes is best.

Faith Over Failure

When the doctors told me I was a good candidate for a kidney transplant, I never doubted I would succeed. Given my age and that I would become a first-time father at forty-four years old, I believed God would enable me to maintain good health and raise that child. Not only did my faith overcome any fear of failure, but I fathered my second child the following year. At that point, I knew that the God I served would not leave my children fatherless.

During my second kidney transplant, God took me down different roads to reach my final destination. Nonetheless, I pushed past those hindrances and ran the race laid before me (Hebrews 12:13). Today, I have two beautiful daughters that are in middle school. I believe that for the rest of my lifetime, I will be healthy enough to care for my children and walk them down the aisle one day. Part of my diligence is to remain faithful and not lose sight of my goal: prolonged health.

The Marathon Continues

I haven't faced many physical challenges following my second surgery. And thankfully, the likelihood of a third transplant is not in sight at this time. My lab work and numbers are the same or better than the day I stepped out of that hospital in February 2018. Given that I have had not one but two kidney transplants, I know that every day is a new day.

I also know that I could be exposed to a virus at any time, and my body could reject my kidney. The effects of that virus could spiral negatively within a short time. Due to this reality, I diligently protect my gift by doing whatever is necessary to keep myself out of harm's way. I adhere to medical guidelines and ongoing pandemic protocols to stay the course during this marathon. As a result, I am healthier today than I was pre-transplant because I'm very in tune with my vitals, diet, and exercise routine.

In conclusion, securing an organ because of a chronic illness is a marathon for which I had to pace myself. My family was quickly eliminated as potential donor candidates when I started this process. Many of my maternal family members had kidney disease. The paternal side of my family was aging and already had health issues. The search process taught me to pivot quickly and never stop fighting for results.

Chapter 13

TRIUMPH AND
VICTORY MINDSET

To proceed on my recipient journey, I had to develop a triumph and victory mindset. Likewise, I believed in the impossible during my first and second transplants because of my relationship with God. Many Scriptures supported my beliefs and were sources of hope during my transitions. My kidney transplant operations never guaranteed a lifetime of healing; instead, they gave me hope to live another day.

Leading Example

I adopted a victorious state of mind because I believe in God's promises to His people. I have seen evidence of His goodness in my life (and others) on several occasions as I navigated the hurdles of being a kidney transplant patient.

Specifically, I had the opportunity to witness my mother outlive her doctor's initial expectations. Not that the doctor's placed a timeline on her life expectancy, but they could not believe she was functioning so well despite medical reports that would support the contrary. She walked, attended events, and lived her life as though she had no illness for quite some time. She had been in and out of the hospital due to several operations, yet she was still maintaining her vitality. The doctors monitoring my mother could not understand her progress.

My mother had the opportunity to attend her fiftieth college class reunion, celebrate fifty years as a member of her sorority Delta Sigma Theta, Inc. (DST), and celebrate the centennial of the DST sorority before her passing. I believe that her consistent prayer life and uncompromisable faith made a difference in how she lived. God blessed her to live as long as she did, and I am grateful for the time I was able to share with her. I will discuss more about how my mother impacted me in an upcoming chapter.

Health Scare

I did not develop a triumphant, victorious mindset overnight. In fact, I faced multiple health scares throughout my transplant journey. One incident occurred in the spring of 2016 when my wife taught a class in the Caribbean. My children and I accompanied her on this business trip, and almost from the beginning, I began to feel ill. I couldn't understand how it was 85 to 90 degrees outside, but I was shivering, had the chills, and could not hold down my food—it was running right through me.

One morning, my children and I went to get breakfast. First, I got my daughters (who were six and seven years old at the time) settled at our table with their food. Then, I went back to the line to pick up my food. As I was bringing my food back to the table, I fainted and then collapsed. I laid there prostrate on my back, unconscious, with two little girls who were scared to death over my condition—they thought I was dead.

Fortunately, personnel at the hotel and guests I had become acquainted with during our stay reached out to my wife for assistance. From there, I was taken to the hospital by ambulance. The medical team conducted a thorough examination whereby they ran scans on my head for signs of a concussion. They also checked me for signs of a stroke. The lab work confirmed I was dehydrated, anemic, and my creatinine level was rising. In other words, my kidney functionality was declining. This was a disappointing revelation.

I thought to myself, "What a way to spend a few days off work and hamper my children's vacation!" Though I never fully recovered, and the incident contributed to the decline of my kidney functionality, God's hand was still on me.

Laugh to Keep From Crying

The way God provided me two kidneys for two transplants confirms that He was (and is) always in control. Although I did everything in my power to secure donors on my own, it was God who orchestrated my surgeries. He provided the donors, nurses, medical specialists, and doctors to perform both transplants at the right time. Though some obstacles and hurdles had to be overcome, God healed me in His time.

I believe God has a sense of humor because He didn't let me determine how I would receive my kidneys. My first donor was a longtime friend, and my second donor was a deceased young man that was my sister's friend's son. Receiving these donations meant that I had to trust Him to deliver the results I needed. What helped me get through both transplants was the peace of knowing that God's fingerprints were all over the process from start to finish.

The name of my first kidney donor is William "Tony" Snoddy. We met in college through mutual friends. When I shared my health challenges with Tony, he did not hesitate to get tested for compatibility. It was a blessing that he was a match. He was a significant reason my first kidney transplant was a success—Tony was essential in extending my life.

Before and after our recovery from surgery, I can recall Tony and me sharing many laughs. He was excellent at making light of difficult situations, most times with a joke. One memory I have was when the two of us were sitting in the waiting room at Johns Hopkins Hopkins. We were there to have some final tests run a few days before surgery.

On that day, my parents accompanied me to the hospital. At that time, Tony began to joke with me, "Here you are, a forty-something-year-old man, bringing your parents to the doctor's office with you! Did you really need to bring your mommy and daddy to the hospital?" His comment was right on time and so, so funny. I remember laughing so hard that I almost fell out of my seat! That instance was just one way Tony and I laughed before knowing the pain we would feel a few days after surgery.

I found it harder to laugh at my pain during my second transplant. I didn't have much of a sense of humor because I was sicker the second time around. In addition, I received my second kidney from a deceased person, so the experience was much more humbling. I was compassionate towards the family for their loss and grateful they had selected me for a direct donation.

Even though I had never met the family responsible for my second donation, God used the organ of a stranger to generate my blessing. This young man had been ill and was fighting for his life. When his parents learned that their son would not survive, they reached out to their inner circle of friends to see if they knew anyone who needed an organ. The parents took this course of action because the young man was registered as an organ donor.

I am forever grateful for the act of kindness shown by this family. Watching how they instilled this benevolence in their son at such a young age—the importance of donating one's organs after passing—speaks volumes about them as parents.

Fortunately for me, my sister and brother-in-law had a good relationship with the family, and they were able to facilitate securing this gift on Valentine's Day. I believe that my connection to this family was by no means coincidental. I had been praying for a kidney for over a year, and the opportunity presented itself when I least expected it. I will never forget their generosity during my time of need, and I appreciate that we were able to stay in contact following my transplant.

Winner's Mindset

The medical professionals at Johns Hopkins encouraged my recovery through a coach's lens. They would say things like, "Hey! You need to get out of bed and walk!" Once I started walking, they would say, "You can do it. You are doing well, Mr. Works. Keep going." In some respects, they treated me as if I was doing physical therapy and trying to get me back on the court—like I was an athlete. I was encouraged to stay active despite my apprehensions because the medical staff helped instill a winner's mindset in me. They taught me to never give up until I reached my desired results.

The hospital surrounded me with great resources and a medical staff that looked out for my best interest. Recovering from surgery in a healthy environment made all the difference. The positive reinforcement pushed me to walk further and longer each day, which in turn, accelerated the process of my discharge and recovery. I have nothing but good things to say about the support and service I received at The Johns Hopkins Hospital in Baltimore, Maryland. Furthermore, I recommend that all patients considering surgery research the hospital that will conduct their operation. In doing so, patients will be able to manage their expectations better.

Pressing Forward

My testimony and what I have witnessed in others have solidified my faith in God—not man. I've recognized God's supernatural powers in action through the many interpersonal relationships in my life. It has been almost twenty years since my PKD diagnosis. Today, I can sit back confidently and talk about the disease that has touched every person in my family. I am more encouraged to share my story because I have evidence of God's goodness in my life.

Although I eventually underwent two transplants, I trusted God's process and appreciated how He rerouted my medical conditions. There is no way I could have become a double kidney recipient without God. I've learned over time to relinquish control over my life and submit to His authority; I've learned to laugh in the presence of my enemies because I know that God has a plan for me to prosper.

As long as I am walking this path, there is no one else I would want to be on this journey with than GOD. I've learned to never lose hope, even amid despair. Trials have also helped lay the foundation of my unwavering faith. I know that God will never fail me because I've had too many successful experiences with Him. When I am able to encourage others to endure, I always do so because I believe that God is still in the miracle-making business.

In conclusion, many factors have contributed to my triumphant and victorious mindset. I have witnessed God supersede for others, including some of my family members who have overcome physical ailments despite logic. Furthermore, I am living proof that God is working miracles daily. My doctors couldn't have anticipated all my blessings because sometimes there were no scientific answers. Science could not explain God's mercy and grace.

I could never have orchestrated the relationships and resources I needed to experience two successful transplants. These encounters were divinely driven. All I did was have faith, trust God, and exhibit patience during the process. I thank God daily because He healed me and taught me to lean on Him for understanding.

My relationship with God helped me press forward, and I have seen the same truth ring loudly for others. Although many people do not feel comfortable sharing their testimony (at least not at first), it is essential to recognize that there is a higher power looking after our wellbeing. God can carry our burdens if we submit to His will. He has made a difference in my life, and I know He can do the same for you. The Lord was with me during my trials and comforted me with a strong support team. As you will learn in the next chapter, I didn't have to face my health crisis alone because…faith has friends.

Chapter 14

FAITH HAS FRIENDS

The only thing more horrifying than facing a crisis is facing it alone. During my transplants, my support system directly influenced my faith—they encouraged me to rely on Christ for peace and understanding.

In the same way, let's consider a group of men who got their paralytic comrade to Jesus by lowering him through the roof (Mark 2:1–12). This story illustrates that good friends are a pathway to faith and life by helping push you past anxiety and fear in dire situations. Let me give you a quick recap if you are unfamiliar with the story. Four friends decided that they needed to help another friend get to Jesus. The men decided that nothing (even the crowds of people blocking the door) would deter them from getting their friend to Jesus for healing. After successfully navigating the paralyzed man in front of Jesus, the sick man was able to secure his healing.

There are so many facets of that story that inspire and intrigue me. First, I love that even though their friend could not perform regular activities due to his handicapped state, they did not stop hanging out with him or give up on him. Most importantly, they carried him along the part of the journey that he could not do on his own. Friends like these are difficult to find and important to keep.

Similarly, my friends, family, medical staff, and countless others impacted me on my spiritual journey. Between their prayers, the giving of their time, and their financial support, I learned that I was not on this transplant road alone. Ultimately, having friends I could count on made dealing with my trials much easier.

My Kidney Coach

Fortunately or not, PKD runs in my family—it's a hereditary disease. Though I was shocked when I initially learned that I had PKD, I have never felt alone in my health journey. My mother was a model kidney patient, and her demeanor was always positive. You would have never known what she was experiencing by the look on her face or what she chose to discuss—she never once complained. I never heard her utter, "Woe is me."

My mom lived her life to the fullest. She and my father traveled, attended class reunions and conferences, and participated in various activities. Her medical team loved her because she gave back as much love as she received. My mother followed the doctor's orders and recommendations as though they were the Gospel.

Nancy Works was the best coach and friend I could ever have. She especially helped me during the initial stages of the transplant process. I observed how my mother approached securing a kidney: she adjusted to dialysis and dietary restrictions, diligently consumed her medications, established new eating habits, and transformed into a "health soldier." She unselfishly passed her knowledge down to me, and I, in return, am passing it down to others.

In mentioning the impact my mother made on me, I can't forget who was cheering her on the loudest. My father stood by my mother's side as her protector throughout the process. Dutifully, he drove her to the hospital for dialysis treatments. He also stayed while the treatments were being administered (four hours per treatment, three days a week). What is more, he picked up food for my mom while she was being serviced and lovingly waited on her hand and foot. He loved her unconditionally, and it was clear that she was his queen!

Additionally, Nancy Works' coaching encouraged me to handle my transplant battle with diligence. As a result, I maintained a daily regimen of taking my medications, attending doctor's appointments, getting my lab work drawn monthly (or bi-monthly), and consistently managing my diet. I credit my mother, my loving coach, who showed me that my body is a holy temple. Romans 12:1, NIV, further confirms, "...that you present your bodies as a living sacrifice, holy, acceptable to God, which is your reasonable service." Her coaching laid a strong foundation for me to abide by, and I miss her more than words can express.

A Friend and a Brother

In addition to my mother, during my kidney transplant journey, I had a good friend who coached me through the process. He, too, had experienced multiple kidney transplants. This friend was a valuable sounding board.

For example, he informed me of recent improvements in medicine and technology. He saw modern medicine's strides made over the past twenty-five years and shared how the experience impacted him. I keenly listened as he divulged his approach to securing a donor. I was numb upon learning that I needed a kidney until I heard his testimony.

My friend discussed the side effects of medications and when to put pressure on the doctors for change. To illustrate, at one point after my transplant, I lost almost 30 pounds. This loss resulted from an adverse reaction to one of my medications. After some discussion, I learned that my friend also had an adverse reaction to the same medication. Our similar experiences were the perfect examples to convince my doctors that my medication needed to be adjusted.

My friend shared the major takeaway that I had to be intentional when speaking with my medical team. In addition, he conducted an exercise with me to let me know where I fit into the big picture with my family (given my health situation). He shared with me that during this time, my priorities should be in the following order:

1. God
2. Greg (this may appear to be strange, but if there is no Greg, there is no family; I need to take care of myself so that I can be there for them)
3. Family
4. Job/employer

Overall, I valued his feedback and learned a lot from his testimony. My hope is that after reading this book, my story will do the same for you.

My Prayer Partner

Considering the severity of my illness, my relationships with others taught me that faith has friends. Though some people treated me differently and, in many respects, abandoned me during my time of need, there was one friend that stood by me throughout my trials. That friend was my dedicated prayer partner, Vaughn Johnson.

In the early 2000s, long before I knew I had kidney issues, I was invited to join a ministry. Brothers in Discipleship (BID) at my church, First Baptist Church of Glenarden, will always hold a special place in my heart. Locally known, BID is a dedicated, three-year discipleship ministry at my church. As part of the program, the "brothers" were told to select prayer partners. The gentleman I was paired with was Vaughn.

Within this ministry, participants engaged in a Christian curriculum. This entailed systematic discipleship study, relationship building, and active participation in ministry outreach. Some examples of our community service included: feeding the homeless, sharing the Gospel through "street witnessing," volunteering at soup kitchens or participating in prison ministry. We performed these acts of service while learning to share the Bible with family, friends, and strangers. After three years, the male participants graduated from the program (myself and Vaughn included).

Every year, the ministry comprises approximately sixty to seventy men to "do life together". Over time, they become a tight-knit group of like-minded believers that expand their faith and spiritual gifts. About twenty-five to thirty men are invited to join the ministry each year. The men are split into multiple groups of eight to ten and are led by a facilitator and co-facilitator. The information shared in this group is confidential and does not leave the safe space. As a result, the brothers in that group develop a strong bond and become close.

Vaughn was about ten years older than I, and in many regards, we appeared to be more different than we were alike (or so I thought). At the time, I was married with no kids; he was single and a father to three children through a previous marriage. We worked in two different worlds occupationally, but most importantly, we both loved the Lord and bonded as spiritual brothers. Vaughn was the perfect prayer partner for me. He had been to places I was trying to go, and truthfully, he may have been getting the short end of the deal as he was more spiritually seasoned than I.

Over the years, amid my health discoveries, I lost touch with Vaughn. However, as God would have it, it wasn't long after that we ran into each other one day and began to talk. At that moment, I began to remember that there was something different about my relationship with him. I realized how much I missed my valuable conversations with Vaughn.

As we reconnected, we discussed the need to get back involved in the brothers' frequent prayer calls. I fully supported this decision because I was really struggling at the time with all the balls I had in the air: work challenges, a child on the way, a pending transplant, as well as how to execute it all at once. During that run-in, we decided we would start by praying at least three times a week. Our prayers proved to be fruitful. Sometimes we would be on our way to work, praying for our families, different work situations, and my urgent need to secure a kidney donor.

Leaning on Vaughn for prayer made me appreciate that I had a brother I could walk with, talk with, and really get poured into while I poured into him. Our friendship journey was significant because we could discuss anything, and the discussions were always bilateral—we both benefited from them. Of course, my kidney need was a considerable part of our prayer list. Still, we also prayed for Vaughn's family, including his adult children and grandchildren.

Vaughn and I bombarded Heaven with the belief that it was not a question of *whether* I would get a kidney; it was just a matter of *when*. We knew it would happen eventually and believed I would be healed. With the complexities of my medical situation, it was comforting to have the ability to talk to someone—that fact alone was reassuring. To this day, we truly have a valuable relationship, and I am grateful for his support.

The Power of Friendship

Regarding the powerful effects of my friendship with Vaughn and many others, I am reminded of the Bible reference regarding the power of two or more coming together in God's name and submitting their prayers. I am a witness that when two or more gather in His name, it will be done. Therefore, it is better for two to pray together for the same thing because there is power in agreement.

My prayer partner Vaughn was not the only one praying for me during my transplant journey. I was stunned by the number of people that I discovered were interceding on my behalf. People I had not seen in years had been lifting me up in prayer; many of these people I was unaware knew about my illness. While recovering from my kidney transplants, I was reminded that I had a deep pool of friends and relationships across the country. I had a host of people talking to God about me, including family, friends from college, church, former roommates, and their spouses.

I was most surprised when I learned that my college roommate from freshman year and his wife, who lived in St. Thomas, U.S. Virgin Islands, had become aware of the health challenge I was battling. When they reached out to me, their support opened my eyes to how God can reconnect His people. Levi and Monique were prayer warriors sending love on my behalf from across the Caribbean. They also had people praying for me that had never laid eyes on me, purely because of my connection to them—now that is humbling. Their encouragement amid others aided me in the fight for my health. Truly, the power of friendship is powerful indeed.

Miracle Granted

My second transplant showed my physical rebuild. Before my transplant, those around me witnessed my physical decline. I lost between thirty to forty pounds over twelve to fifteen months. My clothes were falling off my back. People knew I was sick, but many didn't necessarily recognize the severity of my illness. I'm sure many thought it was cancer, and if I can be transparent, I know there were rumors that I would not survive my complications. Nonetheless, I never hid from my medical situation. I wanted people to see me because I knew that the God I served would heal me eventually.

Imagine the surprise three to twelve months post-transplant when I reemerged looking like a clean bill of health (it was an extraordinary miracle). My evolution was a remarkable example of God's miraculous healing power. I became a walking, talking, breathing testimony of God's goodness. I also learned that God was in control the entire time and that I should never take any of these miracles for granted.

A Loving Spouse

Additionally, I learned that faith fuels a loving partner. My wife, Cynthia, was a true blessing during my journey. As I stated before, she was pregnant with our first child when I first learned I would need to have a kidney transplant. Of course, she could not donate an organ herself, but she coordinated with other family members to see if they were suitable matches. Her initiative was well received.

I also learned that Cynthia sent emails soliciting prayers before my first transplant (which put me on many people's radars). She never mentioned this action to me. Instead, she quietly created a prayer chain of people and allowed the Holy Spirit to move accordingly. I had no idea who was on Cynthia's distribution email chain, but it must've reached hundreds of people. Her faithfulness further signified that many individuals in my corner were rooting for me.

My wife also had her mother fly from Dallas, Texas, to our home in the Washington DC, metropolitan area for support. Her mother stayed with us following my first transplant so that she could help care for our baby and assist Cynthia as she cared for me. Not only did my wife do this, but she also reached out to our network of loved ones after I had undergone the transplant and inspired them to bring us food and nourishment. To this day, we still praise God for those provisions because their responses were phenomenal. Cynthia ensured that no one in our house would have to cook. She was a blessing upon a blessing then, and to this day, she still is.

Faith is a Full-Life Cycle

One of the most amazing things about walking with God is His ability to provide unbelievable experiences that generate comfort and blessing. While undergoing my second transplant, I had an unexpected visitor: a friend whose daughter also had a kidney issue. This person turned out to be one of my parents' closest friends. What is even more remarkable is that more than fifty years ago, this person took care of my mother while she was pregnant with me. What were the odds of me running into her—especially under those conditions? Certainly, this was not a coincidence.

At that moment, I felt the providence of God. I was having a full-life-cycle moment. God had orchestrated this woman (who was my mom's nurse when she gave birth to me) to be present with me once more as I was undergoing my second kidney transplant. I was stunned because I lived forty miles from Baltimore but ended up at Johns Hopkins Hospital during the same interval as her. I repeat this was no coincidence.

I can honestly say that throughout my kidney transplant journey, I have truly had some well-equipped faith friends who have walked through this process with me. Furthermore, I learned along the way that God does not make mistakes. Just like He did with me, when you are in need, He will dispatch a faith community around. When He does, embrace them because they will help you endure your trials and further your testimony for His glory.

Chapter 15

MAKING A GOOD CONFESSION

N ow that you have gotten to know me better, it is time for me to encourage you in whatever battle you are facing in your life. In this chapter, you will gain additional insight on how to use your faith as a weapon against the enemy.

Using Declarations to Jumpstart Your Prayer Life

Declarations are an excellent reminder of the blessings we already have. For this next step, I would like for you to read these bold-print statements out loud:

- I choose to walk by faith and not by sight; I will overcome every obstacle I face regardless of what I have been through.
- I choose faith over fear; I am confident that I will see the goodness of the Lord in the land of the living.

- Not only do I have strong faith, but I also have long faith; my faith will endure.
- I refuse to become weary in my well-doing because I believe I am on the edge of receiving my harvest; I will not faint!
- When I am weak, I will not lean on my understanding; instead, I will lean on God as the Author and Finisher of my faith.
- I will not become stressed or depressed about who leaves my life because God will never leave or forsake me!
- I will not allow my faith to wither because I have been young, but now I am old; however, I have never seen the righteous forsaken nor His seed begging for bread.
- I am an overcomer, and I know that no matter what battle I may face, the battle is not mine; it is the Lord's. Therefore, the fight is fixed, and I am already victorious!

I will say "Amen," as a sign of agreement that those statements will come alive in your heart, mind, soul, and spirit. As found in Scripture, life and death are in the power of the tongue (Proverbs 18:21). I asked you to read those affirmations because I believe that words have power. Therefore, to live a victorious life, you must start by manifesting the favor you already possess.

Prayer Development

You will find that declarations such as those above greatly develop your prayer life. Prayer is the leading resource I use to place my cares, challenges, and trials into God's competent hands. I am not telling you anything I have not experienced. So often, when difficult situations come our way, we are unprepared because our faith is not strong enough to counteract the opposing challenges we face. I realized early on during my sickness that, for whatever reason, God chose me to go through this trial. I also learned I should not attempt to carry this weight or lift this burden alone.

Naturally, some people who experience organ failure pray for a donor. Likewise, I prayed for this and that God would help my body accept the organ. Remember, there is always a possibility of rejection when something foreign is inserted into the body. Before my transplants, I prayed that there would be no rejection from my new organ. I also prayed for minimal side effects to the medication and that I would be able to digest the dosages prescribed because that ensured the most protection for my kidney.

Often, I pray for people nationwide that donate kidneys. I ask God to give them a double blessing for their generosity. For my donor, Tony, I prayed that God would bless him with a family. Within the first couple of years, after I had my first transplant, Tony had not one but two children. I pray that God blesses donors because they sacrifice their organ(s) to provide life-giving opportunities for others.

I am a witness to the power of prayer. I've sat back and watched how God has made impossible things happen; I've seen His supernatural abilities in action. I believe that God grants favor to those who reach out and touch other people, which is why I do my best to bless others, especially during these uncertain times.

Similarly, we can experience significant developments in our prayer life when we entrust God with our burdens. When we are transparent with Him about our needs, He hears us and responds accordingly. He cares about what we are going through and wants to have a relationship with us, but we have to use our free will to accept His assistance.

Faith Expansion

As my prayer life has developed, I have seen my faith expand. The benefits of having a solid relationship with God are endless. Through Scripture reading, I have learned the importance of fellowshipping with like-minded believers—God's children. Consequently, I do not shy away from people who want to help me or learn from my story.

During my transplants, I began looking at my situation as if I were going to the gym. For example, in the gym, all kinds of people work out. Some people are there under protest: they are only compliant because their doctor told them to exercise so that it may help their body fight off disease. Other people are there because they fear their spouse or significant other may lose interest in them if they do not drop a few pounds.

People in these predicaments are generally unable to lift their body weight or handle their relationship problems. Some people are referred to as "gym rats." The term means that they love fitness, are obsessed with the perfect physique, and may be present or former athletes. Whether you are the athletic type or not, one of the most important things to know while exercising is not knowing what you *can* do but what you *should* or *should not* do.

I'll illustrate another example: just because you can lift one hundred pounds does not mean you should. The important thing when exercising is to use proper technique and form. Further performance can lead to severe injuries if your technique is wrong. In the same way, I believe God sends trainers, such as pastors or prayer partners, into our lives to help us develop faith muscles. Faith comes by hearing, and hearing comes through the Word of God. I further believe that the trials in our life work our faith muscles and that, over time, our faith expands and grows. One of the tools that increases that faith is prayer.

Prayer is like a powerful GPS. It allows God to orchestrate your steps. The benefit of a strong prayer life is that it provides comfort when you don't know the direction to travel. To continue our GPS analogy, imagine that you're driving to a destination. There may be many ways to get to your destination; however, you might not necessarily know the best route. Remember that most GPS systems in your car need to be online to access directions. The online connection is key because you may not know or have a degree of certainty of where you are supposed to be going.

Similarly, your faith must be connected to the Spirit of God, who dwells in you. Romans 8:26, ESV reads: "In the same way, the Spirit helps us in our weakness. We do not know what we ought to pray for, but the Spirit himself intercedes for us through wordless groans." This Scripture means that even when you do not know what to pray for, your spirit-being can connect with your Heavenly Father to receive the directions you need for your present journey. God knows what you need to pray for and can deliver it to you before you even ask. That Godly foreknowledge should be good news for you because as long as God is navigating that journey, you will get there the way you are supposed to.

Weighty Concerns

During my transplant journey, I must admit that there was a time when I was utterly overwhelmed. Looking back, I couldn't have endured that season of life without the prayers that kept my faith activated and alive. I recall that I was distraught over the cost of my transplant amidst the danger of my employer filing for bankruptcy. If the company failed, that would place a significant financial burden on me because I would have to pay for the surgery out-of-pocket due to the loss of my benefits. This was an outcome I could simply not afford.

Ultimately, these were weighty concerns that plagued my mind. Instead of burdening myself with worry, I decided to take control of my thoughts and hold myself mentally accountable. To help me cope, I began to look at my situation as a business problem. I segmented the obstacles and began to tackle them one at a time. Honestly, that strategy was the key for me. Attempting to address all my complications at once was challenging and too much to handle. Therefore, I had to take one step at a time.

Prayer-partner Power

Enduring my transplants and the challenges that presented themselves along the way taught me the power of having a prayer partner. As I mentioned, my prayer partner and I tried to pray together daily. We were only briefly successful with that good intention, but we prayed at least three times a week before my prayer partner went to work. By that time, I had stopped working, but the prayers weren't only for my benefit; we were praying for him and all the things he was going through.

Finally, I believe that having more people praying on your behalf helps carry the load forward. Praying creates a mutually advantageous situation for both prayer partners. Proverbs 11:25 NIV further illustrates that "A generous person will prosper; whoever refreshes others will be refreshed." This verse has rung true throughout my life and especially during my health woes.

I also refer to prayer partners as "faith friends." Faith friends are dedicated to helping you see life through the lens of faith. These spiritual warriors are essential to have in your corner when you are believing in a significant breakthrough of any kind. If you don't already have one, I encourage you to pray and seek an accountability partner to do life with—you won't regret it!

Facing Giants

The older I get, the more I realize that faith is not genuine until it has been tried and tested. You cannot move into the next phase of life until you pass the trials that have come before you. I believe that many people stay stuck in life because they cannot overcome the hurt that they've experienced in the past. These challenges will continue to present themselves until these people confront their pain and ask God for the strength to move forward.

Similarly, I am speaking for myself when I say that I don't want to continue making the same mistakes and repeating the same test repeatedly. I am determined to fight these battles with my faith, and I want to encourage you to do the same.

One Biblical character who had great faith combined with outstanding preparation was David. As a shepherd boy, David killed both a lion and a bear. When the giant Goliath stood defiantly against the God of Israel, David's faith propelled him forward to fight. Warding off predators was a part of David's role as a shepherd.

I suspect that the reason for David's preparatory struggles became apparent when he was destined to confront Goliath. David realized that what he experienced in his past was practice for this giant-fighting moment—God was preparing him for a bigger mission. David would have never been equipped to go from the pasture to the palace without first defeating the lions.

Maybe you are facing a giant right now. If so, I want you to be inspired. I always find inspiration in the David and Goliath story no matter how many times I read it. Just as David won a victory against long odds, I won a victory against kidney disease (twice), and so can you!

Remember that David looked small, weak, and meager standing next to Goliath. He was considered feeble and defenseless compared to the larger, mightier fellow warriors. However, David was more prepared for battle and buttressed by faith than any of Saul's senior warriors. In the end, fighting with faith enabled David to win the biggest battle of his life.

Just in case you are new to the Bible or unfamiliar with this story, I want to recap a few significant details. First, on the day of the "moment of truth" confrontation, David decided he was going to fight the giant. Not just any giant, but a giant with experience battling since his youth. Once David made this decision, he prepared for battle. Then he went to a nearby stream and selected five stones for his fight with Goliath.

David could have gathered a single stone, but he didn't; he was prepared to miss. As David walked out for battle, he did not walk out with armor from head to toe. For he knew that if he did, he would be weighed down and unable to move as effectively as possible. Instead, he walked out in the garb he wore as a shepherd boy with a slingshot and five stones. During the battle, David slew the Philistine with one shot. This story is one of my all-time favorites because David, as the underdog, came out, slew the giant, and was victorious despite his "underdog" circumstances!

Likewise, you may have at least one challenge you are facing. Would you like to acquire the spiritual "giant-slaying" asset and add it to your Christian resume? If so, I encourage you to ask God for faith and preparation to fight your giants.

While kidney disease may not seem as massive as Goliath to some, it was a giant for me. It was so big and overwhelming that I was not sure how I would experience victory on the other side of this tremendous obstacle. There were so many things going on simultaneously that I couldn't keep up with all the changes. Nevertheless, I was advised that God is no respecter of persons. I believe that the same way He made a way for me, He can absolutely do the same for you. I believe that by the time you finish reading this book, you will experience a miracle. I believe that you will be ready to embrace a life of triumph after fighting relentlessly for your victory.

As amazing as God has been to me, I believe that He will do even more for you. This belief causes me to roll up my sleeves and fight by getting on my knees in prayer. Prayer is the language of faith: when used properly, it causes favor to manifest miraculously on the Earth.

I believe that when preparation meets opportunity, favor may be unleashed. That process may be preparing you for your transplant by eating a healthy diet, exercising regularly, and waiting patiently. You never know! One night, you might get a call from a donor coordinator at the hospital saying, "We have matched a kidney for you. We need you to come to the hospital immediately so that we can perform the operation tomorrow at 8:00 am." In that case, you must be ready for that call.

When faith connects with favor, that connection creates a move of God so powerful that everyone will know that God, and only God, can move in this way. I believe God is using the situation you are experiencing right now to unlock an unflagging, fighting faith that will defeat every giant you are facing. Therefore, make your declarations, find your prayer partner, and get ready to see your faith come alive in a powerful and new way!

Chapter 16

DO YOUR PART: FOLLOW INSTRUCTIONS

As a kidney recipient, there were many times that I was tempted not to follow my doctor's orders. For example, I was initially disappointed when instructed to change my diet and avoid eating some of my favorite (unhealthy) foods. However, I knew that my doctor had my best interests at heart. Following his recommendations would aid in my speedy recovery. At that point, I decided to lay aside my selfish desires and adhere to healthier alternatives. I don't regret my decision then or now. I am in better physical condition today because I choose to do my part and obey my medical leaders. If you can relate to my circumstances, continue reading for inspiration on how to *do your part* on your health journey.

Obedience is Key

One of the most difficult parts of parenting, teaching, or babysitting is getting children to follow directions. If you have children, cousins, nieces, nephews, or work in childcare, I am sure you can agree. Even with the most straightforward and beneficial instructions, some children are determined to be defiant and ignore authority. This degree of stubbornness can be particularly destructive in any age group. For instance, adults are also susceptible to disobedience.

As a believer, I am reminded of all the times in the Bible when I read that God's blessings were conditionally based upon obedience. To illustrate, God's favor blessed Adam and Eve until they disobeyed God's rule about not eating from the forbidden tree. Abraham did not gain his descendants (that would outnumber the stars in the sky) until he first left his father's land and set out for a land that God would reveal to him.

Both parties were given choices to obey and made decisions that would impact generations to come. Adam and Eve were responsible for introducing sin to the world; Abraham became the father of many nations. Each of these testimonies teaches us that there are consequences when we don't follow instructions. Therefore, we should avoid such destruction by submitting to God's commandments.

Now, you may wonder how these stories relate to your transplant season. Let me explain: if you do not follow the directions of your medical providers, you can set yourself up for organ failure—or worse, death. Your doctor's orders will be inconvenient at times; they may even be unfavorable. Nonetheless, unless absolutely necessary, it is not your responsibility to question every step of your care and defy your medical plan. In doing so, you could expose yourself to dangerous consequences. Instead, it is better to listen to your provider and follow the guidelines they have set for your safety and development.

Follow Your Blessing

Just like obedience, sometimes you have to be willing to travel for greater opportunities. Your *best* life can be directly linked to a geographic region. However, you will never know what your future holds if you don't first step out of your comfort zone and follow the prospects that may arise.

To demonstrate, in November 2020, my youngest sister Kharon and my nephew Solomon traveled from Dallas, TX, to the Washington Metro area to visit my father for a few weeks. He had recently been diagnosed with cancer, and they wanted to spend some time with him. At the time, Kharon's kidney functionality was declining due to her battle against PKD, and she was seeking donors for a kidney. One morning, she received a call from her medical team in Dallas stating that a kidney had become available for her off the transplant list. The call meant that she would need to travel back to Dallas (in less than eight hours) to begin the kidney transplant process.

In less than three hours, her twin sister, Sharon, and my father helped her purchase two plane tickets, pack her belongings, and get her and my nephew on a plane back to Dallas. In addition, we called our cousin Carmelita. We asked her to drive from her home in Oklahoma City to Dallas (over two hundred miles), pick up my sister and nephew from the airport, and take them to the hospital for Kharon's transplant. What was the likelihood that there would be no traffic, no accidents, and no delays on the highway that would hinder her ability to arrive safely? Not only did my sister arrive safely at the hospital, but she also endured a successful operation.

Carmelita embraced the opportunity to help Kharon. It may have been inconvenient at the moment, but that's what our family does, we help each other in times of need. Just four years prior, she had her own kidney transplant. My cousin's donor had two healthy kidneys. However, her donor decided to have one of her two kidneys removed because it was causing her pain. Fortunately for Carmelita, her donor's pain was her gain. Today, my cousin's kidney is thriving, and she has a newfound appreciation for life. Carmelita's testimony further illustrates why we are blessed when we bless others.

God left no doubt that His fingerprints were all over this experience. No one could have orchestrated these events of identifying a kidney, securing last-minute transportation, and traveling safely—but God. Kharon's situation taught me that, at times, you must be willing to move or shift to get the best possible care for yourself or a loved one.

As mentioned, I experienced a similar encounter when my wife and I sought out John Hopkins Hospital for my transplant surgeries. This hospital was well-known for its qualified medical staff and exemplary healthcare center, so my wife and I desired that I receive my care there. In hindsight, I am so glad we made that decision because my experience at Johns Hopkins Hospital was sensational.

Furthermore, as a person of faith, I believe there is a "God factor" and a "we factor." God has a responsibility to do His part, and we have an obligation to do ours. So, following instructions is essential for successfully navigating an illness or life transition.

Accountability

Doing your part in your medical journey may make you uncomfortable at times, but you must follow instructions. Whether it is doctor's orders, mentor's advice, or most importantly, God's calling, you should listen to the knowledge given to you and respond accordingly.

The beautiful thing about God is that He will meet you wherever your faith level is. When we are responsible with our decisions, it is easier to take accountability for the results. For example, in Matthew 8:2–3, a man with leprosy approached Jesus and declared that if Jesus was willing, He could cure the man of his illness. After hearing this, Jesus reached out to the man and commanded him to "Be clean." At that moment, the man was healed because he believed that God would do so, and the Lord provided for him.

Later in Matthew 8:5, a centurion approached Jesus and asked Him to heal his servant. The main difference is that the centurion's faith was greater, but his spirit was humbler; he felt so unworthy of Jesus' coming to his house that he told Jesus he believed that just the mere "words of Jesus" could heal his servant. Jesus granted the centurion's request instantly because he took initiative.

Yet another example of accountability can be found in Mark 5:21. A ruler named Jairus approached Jesus and begged him to come to his house to heal his daughter. Jesus agreed, but while they were on their way to Jairus' house, a woman who had been bleeding for twelve years reached out and touched the hem of Jesus' garment. Her health was instantly recovered.

Even after Jairus saw this woman receive her healing, he still desired for Jesus to come to his house to heal his daughter. On their way, they received the report that the girl had died. Jesus assured Jairus that everything was going to be alright. They continued to the rulers' house, and Jesus healed the girl. Jairus received his blessing because he was adamant about leading Christ to his needs. His relentless pursuit to heal his daughter and unwavering faith were determining factors in how he was granted his request; he felt accountable for his daughter's recovery, and the Lord did not disappoint him.

In summary, I shared these stories with you to let you know that no matter where your faith is, God will meet you there and do His part—you just have to do yours. In times of sickness, you must take your medication, eat the right foods, and maintain regularly scheduled appointments. You must hold yourself accountable for your recovery. While you may not be able to do the rigorous physical activities that you did pre-diagnosis, you should still do some type of doctor-approved exercise. It is essential for your present and future quality of life to follow your medical provider's instructions. I am a witness that it is not easy, but it is so worth it.

Conclusion

I trust you have benefitted from reading Triumph and the aftermath of my PKD diagnosis. Many steps led to my testimony. Some of them include the following:

1. I discovered I had PKD.
2. I adopted the "new normal" and established healthier alternatives to live by.
3. I secured donors for my transplants.
4. I developed a Kidney Transplant Strategic Plan.
5. I addressed my employer through a Workplace PR Strategy.
6. I embraced the recovery process and accepted my transformation.
7. I navigated a pandemic while experiencing the challenges of having a compromised immune system.
8. I ran the chronic illness marathon and generated a triumph and victory mindset.
9. I accepted the support of faithful friends.
10. I followed my medical instructions.

And most notably, I allowed my faith to be stretched during the process. There is nothing easy about being a two-time kidney transplant recipient. Every day, I face challenges that pose risks to my health. In response to these dangers, I have two options: live my life in fear or by faith. I continue to choose the latter.

It is not impossible to enjoy life while battling a chronic illness. You can still fulfill your dreams and destiny with the proper spiritual tools; these include faith, prayer, and works. If you have learned anything while reading this book, I hope it is this: the battle is not over until God says it is over. By embracing the transitions in life and accepting your setbacks, you can learn to persevere through trials. I endured my medical challenges, and as a result, I believe they made me stronger as a husband, father, son, friend, and child of God. The same outcome is true for you if you align yourself with the Lord and trust the plan He has for you.

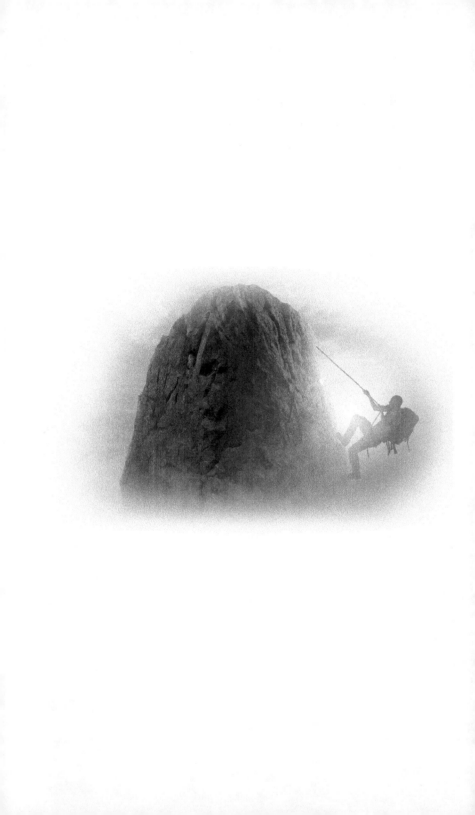

PART 2
DONOR TESTIMONIALS

Chapter 17

BENEVOLENCE: THE GIFT THAT KEEPS GIVING

M*y name is William Snoddy, and I am Greg's first kidney donor. My experience of becoming an organ donor is one that I will never forget and always value. My relationship history with Greg and the seriousness of his health needs aided my decision to help my friend. He faced a medical condition requiring surgery, and I was honored to be of service.*

Relationship History

I met Greg in college many years ago. Although we were not close friends at school, we later discovered that we had much in common. Greg and I had mutual friendships and crossed paths on various occasions. After graduating college, I received a job in New York City and soon learned that Greg was also living there. My roommate at the time was also a friend of Greg's, and they had an active social life. As a result, we hung out together often.

I began to know Greg better and became friends with his roommate. They welcomed me into their circle, and we developed a close bond. For the most part, everyone had something in common with one another. Most of the guys were Morehouse graduates; however, Greg and I were the only two Howard alumni.

Shortly after I moved to New York, Greg and I began to connect, hang out and become good friends. Eventually, we both decided to relocate: Greg went to graduate school in Chicago, and I returned to the Washington, DC, area. Sometime later, I decided to enroll at a law school in North Carolina. Little did I know that Greg would also relocate to NC for a new-found career move. We ran into each other quite a few times. After living in North Carolina, I decided to return to Maryland. Shortly after that move, I discovered that Greg had relocated to his hometown in Silver Spring, Maryland; this was yet another opportunity for us to rekindle our friendship.

Though our various relocations were not intentional, Greg and I somehow managed to stay near each other. As a result, our friendship grew over the years. When we first met, neither of us had any kids. Children were the furthest thing from our minds at twenty and twenty-one years old. Currently, Greg and I are married to attorneys and have two daughters. Coincidentally, my first daughter was born the same year I donated my kidney to Greg. We have more in common now than ever, and I can't stress enough how much I appreciate his loyalty.

A distinct memory of our friendship was when we attended a homecoming football game with his family. Greg's mother used to work at Howard University and was a beloved figure on campus. I was in law school in Chapel Hill, North Carolina, at the time. Greg was living in Winston-Salem, North Carolina. A group of Howard employees and fans (including Greg's parents) drove down to Greensboro, NC, for North Carolina A&T State University's homecoming game against Howard. Greg's family had an extra ticket and graciously invited me to the game. Howard won the game in overtime against one of its most disliked rivals. This event was one of the most incredible live sporting experiences I had ever witnessed. We had a great time.

Situations like these proved to me that Greg was a quality friend. What is more, I grew to love his folks over the years. When Greg asked me to become his donor, I jumped at the opportunity. Donating my kidney to him was not a question of *why* but *when*.

Recipient Approach

I don't vividly remember how I was approached to become Greg's organ donor. I recall a discussion in which he made me aware that he had kidney disease. Later, he asked me to agree to be tested for kidney compatibility. Greg made this request before he knew when he would need a new kidney. I believe he knew that getting a transplant was possible and was trying to get a pulse on whether I would consider getting tested. He phrased the opportunity as one that was contingent on the results of my compatibility. I agreed to be tested because, at that point, there was no immediate surgery date, and I felt that testing for compatibility was the least I could do.

Health Expectations

For me to become a kidney donor, I understood the eligibility requirements to be as follows:

1. The applicant has to be over the age of 18.
2. An applicant with an illness may have the ability to be a donor, but that is contingent on the results of their medical work-up.
3. An applicant must be healthy enough that donating a kidney would not put their health at risk—a donor would need to be able to function with one kidney.

After I met all of these requirements, I donated my kidney to Greg in 2009 (fourteen years ago). I know about the donor process and value the importance of health way more now than I did pre-donation.

Outside of being healthy, there weren't any weight, dietary, or lifestyle requirements that affected my being a good candidate. The medical staff wanted to ensure that I didn't have high blood pressure or any underlying conditions that could affect my health post-donation. Having high blood pressure affects kidney function and could cause other health-related problems. If I had high blood pressure, it is unlikely that I would have been eligible to donate.

At the time, I wasn't doing anything that would cause my body harm. I didn't smoke or drink alcohol. I had excellent blood pressure. In brief, I didn't have any health issues that were serious enough to keep me from the opportunity.

From a mental perspective, the medical staff referred me to a psychologist to ensure that I was mentally prepared to handle the donation process. I passed their screening tests with flying colors.

In addition, I had to go through multiple tests to ensure that I was healthy enough to donate. I recall that I was given a fluid to drink and that a doctor administered me a CT scan afterward. The scan was used to detect any diseases or conditions in my body. I also had to have blood work done regularly. Following all required examinations, I was determined to be the most compatible donor for Greg's surgery.

Decision-making Process

When Greg approached me about donating a kidney to him, the first person I discussed the possibility with was my wife. My wife's response was positive; she fully supported and encouraged my decision to help my friend without hesitation or reservations. She and I both knew that Greg needed this kidney.

This donation was an opportunity to extend the quality of his life, and we were confident that I should accept the challenge. I was already aware of his family history of PKD. I knew the seriousness that could arise from kidney failure, and I felt privileged to help him avoid that misfortune.

Therefore, my decision to support my friend was of good faith and a clear conscience. Our like-minded travels, similarities, and mutual interests had worked out for us to become good friends, so I believed there was divine intervention behind the scenes. With the support of my spouse, I felt reasonably confident in my decision to become a kidney donor.

Once I learned that I was the most compatible source, I knew I could not back out of the opportunity. To my understanding, I was most compatible because my tissues had more matches to Greg's than any other applicant. I was not surprised that so much testing was involved in arriving at this conclusion.

Purpose Driven

Looking back, I do not believe it was a coincidence that Greg and I kept relocating and reconnecting. As I previously mentioned, we seemed to follow one another to the same cities, at the same time, throughout our friendship. I believe God directed our encounters, and it was part of my purpose to serve Greg with my organ. I am a firm believer that God has a prosperous plan for everyone. He already knows our futures and designs situations so that they will work out for our good if we are obedient to Him.

Let's consider what happened with the Biblical character, Joseph. Joseph's brothers put him into a pit hole in the ground. They sold him into slavery simply because they were jealous that their father favored him more. At first, Joseph was probably upset with his brothers for betraying him; later, he recognized their betrayal as divine orchestration. These events were meant to happen because Joseph later became a leader who saved the lives of his people.

Similarly, I don't think Greg and I would have become good friends if I had not moved to New York and reconnected with him. I also don't believe he would have considered me a potential organ donor if we had not maintained contact. Greg and I lived in the same cities and states and hung out while traveling up and down the east coast for various college events. He has always been someone I could count on; he was reliable. I'm glad that our paths crossed several times over the years and that I was able to give back to my friend in his time of need.

Surgery

On the day of surgery, my wife drove me to the hospital very early in the morning. Upon arrival, I was directed into a pre-op room behind a curtain. Next, I was told to remove my clothes and change into the provided hospital garment. From that point, everything was a blur. I was given IVs and anesthesia and woke up in the ICU post-surgery.

In the past, if someone donated or received a kidney, doctors may have cut into their back for best access. However, modern-day medical advancements have afforded doctors a different surgery option for this procedure. For example, during my surgery, I was told that the doctors placed a small hole into my abdomen and expanded it. Then, they used a microscope to examine the area and make an incision. After that step, they pulled my kidney from my groin area. If I had to guess, I'd say there was probably about a three-to-four-inch incision. After the healing process, the incision could barely be seen.

Recovery Process

When I woke up from surgery, I was in excruciating pain—probably the most pain I've ever experienced. When I referenced this to the medical staff, they quickly supplied me with the proper painkiller medication. I was grateful for the meds because, after the dosage, I didn't experience any more discomfort that day.

During my recovery, I was moved into a separate portion of the John Hopkins Hospital. This section was specifically designed for people who didn't utilize insurance. However, it was built more like a luxury hotel. My room came equipped with comfortable sofa chairs and upscale accommodations, such as room service. Upon arrival, I was brought a menu for my wife and me to select our meals. We weren't served regular hospital food; instead, we dined from gourmet selections. It was an incredible experience. The medical staff there truly gave me VIP treatment. I later learned that where I stayed was considered by some as the "donor suite."

The next day, my body responded violently after eating my first solid meal. I could imagine my insides saying, "Hey! Slow down! Something bad has happened here." I began to feel terrible. I remember trying to sleep the rest of that day to no avail. My body reacted unfavorably because a vital part of me, one of my kidneys, had been removed from my body. This was an unusual occurrence, hence the initial pain. While that stage was probably the sickest I have ever felt in my life, the pain and fatigue lasted only twenty-four hours. The following day, I woke up feeling much better. A few hours later, I was discharged from the hospital.

Long-term Aftercare

I took off for approximately four weeks to fully recover from the surgery. In hindsight, I could have returned to work sooner. I took off that time because I didn't know what to expect regarding my healing process.

The medical staff instructed me to return to the hospital a few weeks after the transplant for a post-op follow-up appointment. I was recommended to see my surgeon, Dr. Sege, once or twice for short-term treatment. After the follow-up appointments, Dr. Sege examined my incisions and cleared me for a successful recovery. I was grateful that I was experiencing a smooth road to healing. The most significant part of the process was waiting for the stitches to dissolve.

In addition to short-term care, the hospital wanted me to participate in a donor study. Unfortunately for them, I unintentionally failed to respond to their inquiries. Over time, they stopped reaching out (I'm sure they grew tired of chasing me). I wish I had communicated better with them because I am sure that the participation of organ donors is important to kidney transplant development. If I could go back and do it over again, I would consider being more active in their medical study.

Hypertension

Naturally, I learned a lot about kidney operations as a donor. Specifically, donors with well-controlled blood pressure should not see a decline in their kidney functionality or an increase in their blood pressure. However, over time it is possible to generate hypertension. The results can vary if someone with one kidney develops high blood pressure due to other circumstances. I'm not aware of any health problems caused by being a kidney donor. However, I will say that when a person donates a kidney, that kind gesture automatically places the donor in a kidney disease category.

Nonetheless, a person can still live a normal life with a single kidney. Let me explain: if a person has two kidneys and both work at capacity, they have one hundred percent kidney functionality. But, suppose a person has one healthy kidney. In that case, they have fifty to sixty percent kidney functionality—the single kidney is working at its highest level. This factor was something I didn't realize before I donated, but I have grown to learn more about it over the years.

Finances

Besides my speedy recovery, one of the best outcomes of my donation experience was that it was free. From the beginning of Greg's approach, he assured me that I wouldn't have to come out of pocket for anything; his insurance covered all of my procedures and medical needs. In fact, during my donor surgery, the doctor noticed a growth and decided at that moment to remove it. When I woke up post-op, he informed me of the removal and that I would not be charged for the service. I don't recall what specific type of growth it was. Yet, I was highly grateful for the doctor's initiative—especially since it was at no cost to me.

Life Changes

Since donating my kidney to Greg, my life hasn't changed much. Physically, I feel just as healthy today as I did before the operation. Over the years, I developed high blood pressure (most likely due to genetics), but that was not a result of donating my kidney. This condition developed years after the transplant, and I suspect that my family's medical history of high blood pressure was the main culprit for this onset.

To keep my blood pressure stable and not risk damaging my remaining kidney, I see a nephrologist bi-annually (or every six months). This doctor supplies me with medication to control my blood pressure and pulse and monitor my kidney. Overall, I am grateful health transitions in my life have been manageable.

Present-day Relationship

Greg and I are still close today, but we aren't able to hang out as we did in the past. This infrequency is not because we don't want to. Instead, as fathers of young children, we don't have the same free time as we did when we were younger.

Moreover, the rise of the COVID pandemic has impacted our social lives dramatically. We used to get together and attend sporting or entertainment events frequently. However, that luxury dwindled because of the need for social distancing and quarantine during the Coronavirus pandemic, an international social lockdown.

Family functions and hectic work schedules have also impacted our ability to fellowship. Every once in a while, though, we get together for our children's birthday parties and small gatherings. Greg and I still live relatively close to one another (in the same county), so if a window of free time emerges, we can get together pretty conveniently.

Advice

If I were to advise someone considering becoming an organ donor, I would tell them to do their due diligence in research. Asking the medical providers as many questions as possible will give them the answers they need during their decision-making process. It is also vital to clarify with doctors any misconceptions they may have and what potential risks and complications may occur during and after surgery. Potential organ donors must ask their doctor how their future health will be impacted—especially if they are younger.

When I consider everything I went through to become a donor, I have no regrets about donating my kidney to Greg. In fact, I would do so again. My donation helped Greg obtain a longer, healthier life for nine years. I am grateful I provided that opportunity for him even though the kidney failed sometime later. Despite this failure, God blessed Greg with another kidney; He has been present in Greg's recovery every step of the way.

The next stage of his life has proved to be very promising. I look forward to all that Greg will accomplish in the future through his powerful testimony.

Chapter 18

A SECOND CHANCE

*T*he following excerpt is an interview conducted with the parents of Greg Works second donor. After the passing of their son, Jonathan, Kristen, and Dave Seager felt compelled to donate his organs to an individual in need—Greg was that individual.

Interviewer: What event led your family into this organ donor process?

Dave Seager: Jonathan was 21 years when he passed away from a series of health complications. The doctors believe an accidental overdose of laced fentanyl caused him to choke on his regurgitation.

Kristen Seager: February 4th, 2018, was an extremely traumatic day for our family. Jonathan was lying on his bed in his room when we found him unresponsive. We called the police for help, and medical professionals arrived immediately at our home; they did not try to resuscitate him. Instead, they brought him to the hospital, monitoring his vitals for seven days. The doctor informed us that Jonathan was not making significant progress despite his best efforts. His final test results showed no brain activity. At that point, we had run out of options. We discussed donating some of Jonathan's organs on Thursday, February 8th, with the medical staff. Two days later, he passed away.

Interviewer: What made you two decide to donate your son's organs to someone in need?

Dave Seager: Our family has always supported the organ donor process. When Jonathan first got his license, we encouraged him to register as an organ donor. He agreed because he knew he could benefit others with his body, even in death. Therefore, when the physician informed us that Jonathan's chances of survival were slim due to severe brain damage, we knew we were responsible for the next decision. The reality of our situation was that our son would not survive, but we had a chance to make a difference in someone else's life. Though it was tough, we decided it was best to donate some of his organs.

Interviewer: What was the timeframe given in your decision-making process?

Kristen Seager: I can't recall exactly, but maybe 48 to 72 hours. First, the doctor told us to select which of Jonathan's organs we wanted to donate. Then, we were encouraged to reach out to family and friends to inquire if anyone we knew may need one. Whoever we selected would have to have already been on the organ donor list to be a valid recipient.

Dave Seager: When given these options, we still had a glimmer of hope that Jonathan might recover. However, after considering the odds of his test results, we accepted the reality that he would not survive.

Interviewer: What are some more specifics regarding the recipient selection process?

<u>Kristen Seager</u>: My understanding is that when someone passes away, their loved ones are responsible for directing their organ donations. To be eligible to receive an organ, a recipient must first register on the national organ donor list. We were given two options during this process: select a recipient or allow someone else to choose from the national database. The fact that Dave and I could supersede this list by directing the donation to someone we specifically knew was comforting; ultimately, that was the route we decided to take. If we could not locate prospects, the hospital administrators would select a recipient on our behalf. There was no option to see the list and pick from it because many factors go into the donation process (primarily geography).

<u>Dave Seager</u>: We were given the option to donate Jonathan's entire body but decided against that because we didn't want Jonathan to become a corpse for experimentation in a laboratory. So, we agreed it was okay to take ligaments, tendons, and other viable organs that people could use immediately. Following these removals, we had him cremated. We donated Jonathan's heart, kidneys, and other organs to recipients we knew were in need. Kris and I met Greg through his sister Sharon, and her husband, Bob. Blood type-wise, Greg and Jonathan weren't necessarily compatible. However, the doctors ran enough tests to determine if they would work well together. Jonathan's other kidney recipient was Kris's friend of a friend from New Jersey. This person was also my best friend's cousin's wife (unbeknownst to us). It was just incredible how the donation process worked out for everyone.

<u>Kristen Seager</u>: The silver lining in this process was identifying a recipient in need and making an impact on their behalf. I am grateful that we could ask the people around us if they needed organs first because it made the experience much more personal. It felt good to give back and make a positive difference in a negative situation.

Interviewer: How long did it take for the medical professionals to remove the organs?

Kristen Seager: Only a few days. The medical staff removed Jonathan's organs the same day Greg underwent surgery: Wednesday, February 14th, 2018.

Interviewer: During the decision-making process to donate Jonathan's organs, was there anyone that you all consulted with for support?

Dave Seager: No. We notified our daughters, but that was it.

Kristen Seager: Yeah, it was a decision that we were already confident facilitating.

Interviewer: Were you able to maintain a relationship with the recipients?

Dave Seager: We have stayed in touch with Greg as he received one of Jonathan's kidneys. We are not in contact with the recipient of Jonathan's heart, but at one point, he sent us a letter thanking us for the donation.

Interviewer: What about Mr. Greg specifically helped you two maintain contact and continue your relationship beyond the transplant?

Kristen Seager: As I mentioned, my husband and I were introduced to Greg through his sister Sharon and her husband Bob, with whom we are good friends. Several months following Jonathan's passing, we went to a funeral held coincidentally on Jonathan's birthday, September 22nd. Dave and I decided to go and pay our respects to the family that had lost their teenage daughter to cancer. Later that same day, our parish held an Offering Mass in loving memory of Jonathan. A mutual friend shared details about this special Mass—that would be held in memory of Jonathan and the repose of his soul—with Sharon, and she shared that information with Greg. They both participated in the Offering Mass that day. That was the first time we met Greg as Jonathan's kidney recipient.

Dave Seager: It was a very emotional moment.

Kristen Seager: I believe there was no better way to meet Greg because, at that moment, there was no anticipation or nervousness. Amid our mourning, we showered him with all of our tears. It meant so much to us to see him in person, which solidified our friendship with him. I will never forget how he supported us that day–it was a beautiful encounter.

Interviewer: Were any costs associated with donating organs on your son's behalf?

Dave Seager: No, the hospital took care of everything. I remember we received some bills, but when we called the hospital administrators to discuss them, they told us that we had received them in error. We ultimately had no financial responsibility for facilitating Jonathan's organ donation. I think the hospital even picked up some of the costs associated with Jonathan's care.

Interviewer: What advice would you give someone considering becoming an organ donor or donating organs on behalf of their loved one(s)?

Dave Seager: I would say that even in death, the human body can benefit those with needs here on earth. There is no redemption in being buried with one's organs, so why not give them to someone who can immediately use them? It is a beneficial process for everyone involved.

Interviewer: Would you recommend others in your situation consult with a doctor before agreeing to the organ donor process? For example, did you have reservations about how Jonathan would look post-donation at his funeral service?

Kristen Seager: We were probably going forward with the donation regardless of what the doctor may have said because we had already agreed to do so. However, it was reassuring to hear the doctor's medical perspective. Regarding how Jonathan looked post-donation, the doctors confirmed that they would remove some of his organs and tissues and make the rest of his body look normal. Dave and I appreciated that the surgeon was careful about preserving his likeness. To our relief, during the open casket funeral, Jonathan looked entirely like himself.

Interviewer: How has losing your son and completing the organ donor process affected your relationship as a married couple?

Kristen Seager: It's been an overall positive experience. Donating Jonathan's organs gave life to Greg and a few other recipients. Although we donated some of his organs to different bodies, Dave and I recognize that Jonathan is still biologically present.

Dave Seager: I read many grieving books and concluded that everyone grieves differently. However, one thing Kristen and I have learned and agree on is that John's still with us—in our hearts and minds. We talk about him all the time, and the more we talk about him, the stronger our memories are of him. Whenever I see Greg, the interaction increases my memory of Jonathan. My wife and I were able to prolong Greg's life by donating our son's kidney and extending his time with his family. *That* is a powerful cycle of life.

Interviewer: Is there anything else you two would like to share with readers regarding your experience facilitating Jonathan's donation?

Dave Seager: I have a joke I'd like to share! To relate, you must appreciate the context and have a good sense of humor. Otherwise, you may be offended by the punch line. To give some background, my son Jonathan used to love rap music. He bonded over hip-hop with his friends, one of them being an African American musician from Miami. This friend wrote a song about Jonathan living on the edge and performed it at his funeral. I get teary-eyed just thinking about that incredibly spirited performance. I remember sharing this experience with Greg, and he made a comment I will never forget. I told him, "John had a lot of brothers that loved him." Then Greg responded, "And now, he's *in* a brother!" Considering that Greg is African American, and the term "brother" is commonly used in their culture to describe friends, we got a good laugh from that irony (laughs)!

Kristen Seager: Jonathan was well-loved by so many people. Dave and I are happy that it worked out for Greg to receive his kidney. Ultimately, we are grateful for the lasting friendship the experience has created–that has made all the difference for us!

ABOUT THE AUTHOR

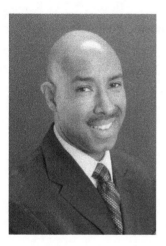

G regory S. Works, "Greg," was born in Ardmore, OK, and raised in the Washington, DC, metropolitan area. He is a two-time kidney transplant survivor. Based on his trials fighting Polycystic Kidney Disease, he is very well-equipped to tell the story of how to overcome adversity to triumph. He does this with a roadmap he developed to be victorious in securing an organ twice for kidney transplants. His story is far-reaching as it provides insight into how to successfully battle a health challenge. The lessons Greg shares can be applied to fighting obstacles on the job, in school, and in sports, to name a few.

Greg has spent the past two decades working as a business development and sales executive for two Fortune 50 Companies and a Big

Four Consulting Firm. He also serves on the Board of Trustees at Lincoln University, PA (HBCU). Greg is a Board Member of the Kids in Need Foundation and Kappa Scholarship Endowment Fund; he lends his financial and investment expertise to these organizations. He is armed with a Bachelor of Business Administration in Accounting from Howard University in Washington, DC, and a Master of Business Administration in Marketing and Finance, from the J.L. Kellogg Graduate School of Management at Northwestern University, in Evanston, IL.

Greg is a member of The First Baptist Church of Glenarden and a servant leader within the men's ministry in the Washington, DC, community. He is a father of two daughters, Kylie and Kelsey, and husband to Cynthia Works.

NOTES & REFERENCES

1. Chapter 1: An Unexpected Discovery
    - Polycystic Kidney Disease
2. Chapter 2: Moving Forward & Establishing Healthy Alternatives
    - Search Gout Symptoms and Treatments – Information on Info.com
    - Chronic Gout Treatment.com
3. Chapter 3: New Beginnings
4. Chapter 5: The Kidney Transplant Strategic Plan
    - The Low Protein Diet for Kidney Disease: Everything You Should Know
        - Recipes & Nutrition
        - Managing Your Diet
5. Chapter 6: Facing the Facts (Workplace PR Strategy)
    - Brown, Brene'. Dare to Lead "Brave Work, Tough Conversations, Whole Hearts.", 2018
6. Chapter 9: Transformation
    - Bible, New King James Version
        - Romans 8:28
7. Chapter 11: Life Forever Changed

- ◆ Treatments
- ▪ Dare To Lead
8. Chapter 12: A Day in the Life of a Kidney Transplant Patient
    - ▪ Holy Bible, New King James Version
        - ◆ Psalm 27:13,14
        - ◆ Hebrews 12:1-3
9. Chapter 14:Faith Has Friends
    - ▪ Holy Bible, New King James Version
        - ◆ Mark 2:1-12
        - ◆ Romans 12:1,2
        - ◆ Matthew 18:19,20
10. Chapter 15: Making a Good Confession
    - ▪ Holy Bible, English Standard Version
        - ◆ Romans 8:26
    - ▪ Holy Bible, New International Version
        - ◆ Proverbs 11:25
    - ▪ Make General Reference to "David & Goliath"
11. Chapter 16: Do Your Part Follow Instructions
    - ▪ Holy Bible, New King James Version
        - ◆ Genesis 3
        - ◆ Genesis 17
        - ◆ Matthew 8:2,3,5
        - ◆ Mark 5:21

A free ebook edition is available with the purchase of this book.

To claim your free ebook edition:

1. Visit MorganJamesBOGO.com
2. Sign your name CLEARLY in the space
3. Complete the form and submit a photo of the entire copyright page
4. You or your friend can download the ebook to your preferred device

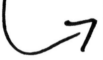

Morgan James
BOGO™

A **FREE** ebook edition is available for you or a friend with the purchase of this print book.

CLEARLY SIGN YOUR NAME ABOVE

Instructions to claim your free ebook edition:
1. Visit MorganJamesBOGO.com
2. Sign your name CLEARLY in the space above
3. Complete the form and submit a photo of this entire page
4. You or your friend can download the ebook to your preferred device

Print & Digital Together Forever.

Snap a photo

Free ebook

Read anywhere

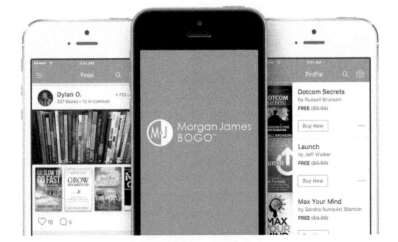

CPSIA information can be obtained
at www.ICGtesting.com
Printed in the USA
JSHW081955170523
41788JS00001BA/8

9 781636 980621